Happy Birthday Eric,
may you have health &
happiness for many
years to come!

Jason Bussel

8/11/09

THE ASIAN DIET

Simple Secrets for Eating Right, Losing Weight, and Being Well

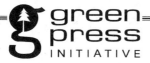

green
press
I N I T I A T I V E

THE ASIAN DIET

Simple Secrets for Eating Right,
Losing Weight, and Being Well

By Jason Bussell, MSOM, L.Ac.

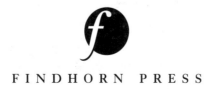

FINDHORN PRESS

First published by Findhorn Press 2009

ISBN: 978-1-84409-160-7

British Library Cataloguing-in-Publication Data.
A catalogue record for this book is available from the British Library.

Edited by Jane Engel
Cover design by Damian Keenan
Layout by Prepress-Solutions.com
Printed and bound in the USA

1 2 3 4 5 6 7 8 9 10 11 12 13 14 13 12 11 10 09

Published by
Findhorn Press
305A The Park,
Findhorn, Forres
Scotland IV36 3TE

t +44(0)1309 690582
f +44(0)131 777 2711
e info@findhornpress.com
www.findhornpress.com

Table of Contents

Preface

Welcome to my book, which I hope you will enjoy. I also hope you learn many things that will help you for the rest of your life.

Have you ever noticed the shape of the average American compared to that of the average Asian? There are more obese people in America than any other country and the problem is growing rapidly. This trend is the result of poor diet and inappropriate lifestyles. Fortunately, we are finally waking up to what the Asian cultures can teach us in terms of health care (acupuncture, herbology, tai chi, etc.); now it is time to learn what they have discovered about eating and living in balance.

The material that is contained in this book is information I try to instill in all my patients. At the onset of treatment, I give them all a talk about adjusting their diet, lifestyle, and attitudes in order to improve their health, mood, and longevity. Many of my patients have asked where they could get this information in written form and as I was unable to find such a resource, I wrote this book.

About me

I am an acupuncturist and herbalist, trained in the United States and I also completed advanced training and an internship in China. I am the President of the Illinois Association of Acupuncture and Oriental Medicine and have a private practice, together with my wife, in Wilmette, Illinois. Many astute people have noticed that I am not Asian and often wonder how can a white guy practice Oriental Medicine?

I earned a bachelor's degree in psychology and worked in psychiatric hospitals for several years before returning to school to study pre-med. As I was applying to med schools, I was dismayed to learn how unhappy the doctors with whom I worked were. I kept hearing "Don't go into medicine. Do anything else. The money is not there, the autonomy's not there, the respect's not there, and even the patient contact isn't there anymore. There's no good reason to be a doctor."

The first 20 times I heard it, I shrugged it off; but I kept hearing it and eventually it got to me. Then a nurse with whom I worked told me about the acupuncture program in town and though I had been interested in Eastern philosophy since taking a course in high school, I had never considered Oriental Medicine (OM) as a career.

I read some books about OM and found the whole paradigm pretty strange and even a little suspect. I come from a family of physicians and was already pre-med myself and I understand things like bacteria and viruses; but the Chinese talk about things like "wind-cold invading the lung" and Qi. It was all so foreign and different and I didn't know if I could ever believe in the system. I figured I could make a living at it because enough other people would believe. My skepticism was very short-lived once I saw how effective this medicine is and how much sense the philosophy makes. Now I love what I do. I get to spend a lot of time with my patients, and I get to help them. In psychiatry, I worked pretty much with a chronic population where very few people ever improved. With Oriental Medicine, I am able to help almost all of my patients safely. Oriental Medicine is the acquired wisdom of thousands of years of experimentation, observation and documentation and with this historical perspective, much has been learned about what works and what doesn't. I am a grateful recipient of these lessons and now I want to share this knowledge to help people take better care of themselves and live longer and happier lives.

I have presented this information with many groups and patients and I know that this system will be difficult for many people to work with at first. This book presents guidelines and suggestions, but it does not tell you what to do. It is up to you to decide how to implement the suggestions and create your diet. The South Beach Diet was so successful partly because it told people exactly what to do. Many of us like being given a strict structure to follow . . . for a while. But after about 60 days we get tired of having no freedom and break from a prescribed regimen. So I am just planting seeds; how they germinate is up to you. And, it is not an all-or-nothing proposition. If you have a bad day, don't give up, start again so you can have more good days.

The opinions expressed in this book are just that – opinions and the book makes no claims to being definitive or authoritative. The principles are written, as I understand them, from my years of studying Oriental Medicine and Asian culture. The ideas come from many different authors, speakers, researchers, teachers, folk teachings, plus my own ideas of what makes sense. Other authors and disciplines may disagree with some or many of the tenets I will present in these pages. Therefore it is up to you, the reader, to decide whether or not this makes sense to you. As far as I know, the Chinese have been studying nutritional therapy longer than anyone else, so I tend to believe that they have figured some things out in the past 4,000 years. The principles are simple:

- Balance and Moderation
- Cooked foods are better than raw
- Vegetables are better than fruit
- White rice is better than brown, but a variety is best
- Diet should be mostly plant-based, with grains and a little of everything else
- Simple foods are better than processed food
- Dairy is not necessary and can be harmful
- Do not over-fill your stomach
- Don't stress too much
- Exercise every day, but not too much
- Keep a wide perspective and don't sweat the small stuff

All these principles will be explained in more detail as you read the book.

What this book is and what it is not.

This is **not** a weight-loss book, but it **is** about getting into balance by eating appropriately. Some of my patients who do not need to lose weight are still very much out of balance. If they are over-weight, that is in itself an imbalance. As you get into balance, you will naturally shed the excess pounds and become more fit. But even those who do not need to lose weight still need this information and **eating right** will prevent or correct all types of disease and disorders. Our diet choices are the most important and influential thing we can do to affect our daily, and long term, functioning.

Chinese Dietary Therapy is a highly developed science and many people spend their whole lives studying and practicing this. There are food cures for all types of ailments, but that is not what this book is about. If you want to learn how to address a certain ailment with diet therapy, please consult *Chinese Nutrition Therapy* by Joerg Kastner and Anika Moje or *Chinese System of Food Cures* by Henry C. Lu (unfortunately out of print but maybe you can find a second-hand copy). There is also a great deal of information about the foods that we commonly eat and how bad they are for us (and I could cite many studies on the subject), but that is not what this book is about either. I present the basic guidelines for eating right and most of us could greatly benefit from these simple changes. If you want to learn what foods to eat to treat a particular disease, or if you want to know everything there is to know about a particular food, read *Healing with Whole Foods* by Paul Pitchford. To learn how we have been misinformed about diet and to peruse many studies on how harmful our standard food choices are, read *The China Study*" by T. Colin Campbell. To learn the basics of eating right and being well, however, read the book you hold in your hands right now.

Acknowledgments

Chinese medicine would be nowhere without building upon the work of others. I would like to thank the entire lineage of Chinese medical practitioners for amassing this wisdom and passing it on; from the Yellow Emperor Huang Di, to Dr. Hui-Yan Cai. I would also like to thank the Midwest College of Oriental Medicine, my alma mater, for educating me and facilitating my study in China. Among the modern-day authors who deserve a lot of the credit for the content of this book are: Henry Lu, Bob Flaws, Kim Barbouin and Rory Freedman, T. Colin Campbell, Joerg Kastner, Anika Mole, Ted Kaptchuk, Dan Bensky, Michael Pollan, and many more. I would also like to thank my family for supporting my career choice, and my wife for making me so much more than I ever was before her.

Chapter One

Introduction to the Asian View on Diet

Asian medicine, like Asian philosophy, is all about balance, that is, finding and maintaining balance as the goal of life. All pathologies can be thought of as some type of imbalance; if you have a fever, you have too much heat; if you have the chills you don't have enough heat. It gets much more complicated than this, but everything can be viewed as too much or too little of something. Oriental Medicine (OM) can help bring a person back to balance. But my greater job as a practitioner of OM is to teach my patients how to live in balance so that they will not need continued treatment. The three greatest factors that get us out of balance are our: Diet, Lifestyle, and Attitudes. The typical Westerner is almost always out of balance in all three areas, sadly and our habits are spreading around the world.

An ancient Chinese doctor once wrote that "In cases of disease and disorder, the physician should first address the diet and lifestyle. If that fails, then you proceed to the more heroic modalities of acupuncture and herbs." Hippocrates, the father of Western medicine wrote, "Let your food be your medicine and your medicine be your food." These days we have lost the sense of connection between what we put in our bodies and how our bodies then function.

Oriental medicine is meant to be a preventive medicine and in the old days it was common to pay the physician on a monthly basis; if, however, you became sick, you would get a refund, for the doctor's job was to keep you healthy, not to help you recover from sickness. If you developed an illness or a disease, the doctor had already failed you. Part and parcel of this agreement was the understanding that the patient would follow the doctor's orders. However, in the West, we are not very good at following our doctor's recommendations. In China they know that if they follow the suggestions, then the problem will not become worse; and if they don't, then the problem will almost certainly progress. Today not enough attention is paid to preventing disease and health disorders; but if we eat right, act right, and think right, we can improve our health for our whole lives. We should all be able to live to 100 years old and not suffer from obesity, heart disease, cancer, arthritis, osteoporosis, Alzheimer's, diabetes, high cholesterol, enlarged prostate, and all the disorders that plague American seniors.

(Some people point out that many Asians do not live to be 100 years old. However, they have other problems such as poor sanitation, parasites, and poverty; and many do not follow the teachings. More and more Asians are embracing the American lifestyle and diet . . . with regrettable results; but if more people followed the principles outlined in this book, many more would reach the century mark.)

The first thing we need to do is change the way you think about food. We have a dangerous disconnect in understanding how the things we put in our bodies affect the way our bodies function. This is partly due to purposeful misinformation in the advertising from the food manufacturers and partly due to our own denial. It is time to take responsibility for your health for you are literally what you eat. Our cells are constantly dying and new ones are being made and those cells are made from the food we eat. If you were to build a house, you would choose to use the best-quality lumber you could find. You will be in your body a lot longer than any external structure, so when you are thinking about what to eat, ask yourself, "What kind of a house am I going to build today?"

We cannot continue to ignore our bodies' needs. Most of us pay more attention to the maintenance needs of our cars than the needs of our bodies. If you put cheap gas in your car and your car starts breaking down, you would change the gas. But, when our bodies break down, we continue to use the same gas. The body's needs are very simple, requiring primarily a plant-based, varied, and mostly cooked diet. There is no magic bullet. **The keys are balance and moderation**.

Western Dietary therapy is still in its infancy, so this is why people keep getting fooled into believing that there **is** a magic bullet. "Everyone should eat granola!" we were told, and then further research showed that too much granola was bad. "Avoid fat and cholesterol and you will prevent heart disease!" but then we found that some types of cholesterol are good and that a low fat diet does not prevent disease. "Eliminate carbohydrates and eat meat to lose weight!" but we learned that this type of diet causes long-term damage to the body. The Chinese have been studying this for thousands of years and have learned that **it is not any one thing that we all need to eat or avoid** – it is finding the proper balance of all things. And they have found that this proper balance can be maintained by eating mostly cooked vegetables, simple grains, plus a little bit of almost everything else.

Let me be clear: there is no one thing that is the key–not fat, calories, sugar, grapefruit, protein, carbs, sodium, trans-fat, supplements, nor any one thing; it is all things and how they combine to form a whole.

Chinese dietary recommendations differ from those that we learn here in the West and some of the recommendations in this book may seem like blasphemy after what you have been taught. I am sorry, but you cannot trust what the government and what your doctors tell you about nutrition. The food industry is thoroughly in bed with the government and makes sure that all dietary recommendations that are released promote their foods. There are conflicts of interest at all levels of the FDA, USDA, National Institute of Health, the Department of Health and Human Services, and the Department of Education. From kindergarten through senior year of high school, most children have two choices for a beverage with their lunch – milk and chocolate milk. And the dairy board gets to decorate the cafeterias with its ads portraying milk as a healthy food. What other industry is allowed such access to directly lobby our children?

And they get to educate our doctors too. In the entire four years in medical school, the average doctor receives just 21 hours of education in nutrition, and the educational materials are often created and provided by the dairy, meat, and snack food industries. What do you suppose these industries want to teach doctors about their products? When scientists stand up to the system and fight for what is right, they are discredited and bullied out of the industry. Doctors are not being evil or negligent, they just tell you what they were taught by those who have products to sell. For example: "Diet does not affect health", "Dairy is good", "Eat a lot of meat", "Supplements can replace whole foods", etc., and the doctors are usually unaware that their education has been provided by special interest groups.

Chinese culture has state-supported health care, so it is in their best interest to teach the people how to be well. In America, health care is a for-profit endeavor and the more sick people there are, the more money there is to be made. I don't mean to sound alarmist or conspiracy-inclined, but it is true; the food and health care industries have so much money and they have tainted the systems that we count on to ensure our safety. You cannot blindly trust their recommendations.

The food choices you make are probably the most influential things you can do to help or hurt yourself on a daily basis. People say they don't have time to cook, or to shop, or prepare good food and they argue that poor nutrition is one of the sacrifices of a modern lifestyle. **We have to make it a priority.** I also hear, "Everything will kill you, so let's enjoy ourselves now." However, **I** plan to enjoy my life for a full 100 years and I don't want to be saddled with excess weight and health problems. Let's face it, eating bad and artificial food is not the only thing we are here to enjoy.

The development of Asian Dietary Therapy

A long time ago, humans found themselves here on this planet. A couple of hours later they found themselves here and hungry, so they started eating things. Then they noticed that different foods affected them in different ways: "That leaf makes me tired, this one make me feel awake; this seed gives me diarrhea, this fruit stops the diarrhea," etc. The real treasure of the Chinese culture is that it is a 4,000 year long experiment with careful record keeping and dissemination of the lessons learned through written language. They never had a Dark Age. Throughout their history, the Chinese have experimented with different dietary and lifestyle choices. When they found things that worked, they spread the word; when they found things that didn't work, they also spread the word. We are the fortunate recipients of the knowledge gained over 4000 years of experimentation, observation, and documentation of the lessons learned by some of the greatest minds in Asia's history. Most of the West's classical knowledge was lost with the fall of the Roman Empire. It is only since the Renaissance that we have started rebuilding our knowledge base, so our knowledge is only about 400 years old.

At its core, Oriental medicine is all about balancing Yin and Yang. This concept will be explained further in Chapter 18, but for now you should know that Yin and Yang is a way of understanding everything in the universe as lying between two extremes: Yin is the cool, quiet, dark energy of things while Yang is the hot, active, light energy. Too much or too little Yin or Yang are forms of imbalance and can manifest as all types of symptoms, including obesity.

You do not need to eat Asian food to follow these principles. In Asian cultures, a great variety of foods, spices, and preparations are included in each country's diet. But there are some commonalities and you can and should adapt these concepts to fit your environment. For instance, look at the way typical Asians behave:

- They eat a lot of grains
- They eat a lot of vegetables
- They don't eat a lot of raw foods
- They don't eat a lot of meat
- The eat a lot of whole foods
- They have few sweets except for a little bit of fruit
- They have soup with most meals
- They have tea with most meals
- They have few baked and processed foods
- They do not consume dairy
- They exercise every day
- They do not get too emotional or stressed

If we incorporate these principles, we will develop the physique of the typical Asian, which is lean. Unfortunately, when Asians come to America and adopt our dietary ways, they develop the shape (and health problems) of the typical American. Diet is more important than genetics in determining our size, shape, mood, health, and longevity.

Don't let your tongue dictate your diet

Food stays on your tongue for one to two minutes but your digestive organs wrestle with that material for 48 hours (normally), and the tissues that are created from that food stay in the body for weeks or months. So the tongue can have a vote, but it shouldn't have the only vote. We all tend to include plenty of sweet and salty tastes in our diet, and sweet has a tendency to create dampness (which is how the Chinese understand excess weight) and salty causes water retention. The Chinese recognize five flavors: sweet, salty, sour, bitter, and acrid. Each flavor has a distinct effect on the individual, and each one corresponds to an internal organ. We have to feed all the organs in our bodies, not just our taste buds. If we don't have enough of all the tastes represented, we will be pulled out of balance.

All foods and herbs have properties and some properties are warming, cooling, moistening, activating, or sedating, etc. Through the considerable study of these properties and the continual recording of results over the centuries, the Chinese have come to understand the actions of food. So, in Asia, the properties of foods are taken into account when planning meals. In addition, there are some foods that are not eaten at certain times because they are contra-indicated; for example, women will not eat cold or raw foods after childbirth because digesting it steals too much of their body energy. Also, some foods are only consumed in certain seasons.

A note about calories: Calorie counting is a flawed concept and I can't believe that no one has pointed this out yet. Calories are different from energy and we want to get all the energy from the food we can and thus we'll then be animated and active and able to burn the calories. But we don't really have to concern ourselves with the calories at all.

In the West, calories in a particular food are determined by burning it in a laboratory with a device called a calorimeter. Then the amount of energy that is released as it is burned is measured. The theory is that the amount of energy released by breaking it down via fire in the lab is the same as would be released by breaking it down with enzymes and digestion in the body. Now these are two very different processes and could most likely yield different results, as many things behave differently in a lab. Even though I'm not convinced that the calorimeter gets a valid assessment of the energy we get from the food, let's assume it is true. So if a bagel has 200 calories worth of energy in the lab, eating that same bagel will put 200 calories into you according to this theory. The thing is, not all of that bagel stays in you. When we move our bowels, we excrete the leftover, unused portion of the food and this has caloric value as well. If we burn the feces, we can measure how many calories we have passed. So the true measure of calories retained would be: calories put in minus calories passed minus calories burned. I am not suggesting that we all start burning our feces; I am just pointing out that the number of calories ingested is not the whole story. For instance, if someone is suffering from dysentery, it doesn't matter how much food they eat, they'll not hold on to any of it. The average Chinese person consumes from 25-40% **more** calories than the average American; even the most sedentary office workers consume more calories and are less obese than we are. You do not need to count calories and you should never go hungry. **The goal here is efficient digestion.**

A key difference between Eastern and Western thought

Western philosophy tends to be reductionistic, i.e., breaking everything down to its smallest parts, while Eastern philosophy is holistic, understanding how things relate to the whole. Each has advantages to offer, but each has limitations. Imagine trying to understand the hand by chopping off the arm and studying the hand alone on a table. It would not make a whole lot of sense without knowing about the muscles and nerves and tendons and blood supply necessary to make it work. Western dietary therapy treats food as nothing more than the sum of its parts, whereas Eastern nutritionists understand that it is how things are combined that matters. So we don't worry about the grams of fat, protein, carbohydrate, sugar, etc., we simply think about the whole food and how it fits into the whole diet.

By the way, it is only recently that we have looked to science to tell us how to eat. Coincidentally, since then we have become more obese and have more diet-related disease. The interactions of complex foods with our complex bodies is much more intricate and involved than we can understand easily. Therefore, we should trust what thousands of years of culture have taught us. We should eat what our mothers and their mothers ate.

Some people say, "Our diet must be OK because we have a longer average lifespan than some countries in Asia". Do not confuse lowered infant mortality and life-prolonging medical care with wellness. We now have more diet-related illness than we have had in the past 200 years.

A note on whole foods

"Whole foods" means using the entire food as opposed to just a single part and this is how the term is used to describe brown rice as a whole food. Oftentimes, one part of a food will have a particular action and the other part will have the opposite reaction. For example, Ephedra stem *encourages* sweating, while Ephedra root *stops* sweating. Citrus fruit *engenders* phlegm and dampness in the body and the peel of a citrus fruit *resolves* phlegm and dampness. I don't expect people to start eating citrus rind, they don't in China either; but you can put it into a tea and absorb its benefits that way. I find the case of grapes very interesting, because for years now, the growers have manipulated the grapes to grow with no seeds. Yet, the main ingredient in antioxidant pills is grape seeds! If we were not taking grape seeds out of our diet, we would not need to put them back in. Every food is balanced and has both Yin and Yang aspects and if we only eat part of a food, we are eating an unbalanced food. This is fine in moderation, but over time our bodies become out of balance.

Whole foods can also refer to an entire part of the plant that is unprocessed. Corn is corn. Corn that is ground down and mixed with soy lecithin, oil, salt, colors, additives etc, is no longer corn and is not a whole food. Nowadays we tend to think (and talk) about a food as nothing more than its constituent parts. "You need some Vitamin C; you should eat more protein, eat less fat, etc." Instead, we should start talking more about the whole foods. "You should have some nuts, you should have an orange, you should eat less meat and dairy, etc." Whole foods are balanced. They are immensely complex and work best when in their whole form.

Fortified foods are foods that have been stripped of their natural nutrients but have had a select few re-introduced. Western, reductionistic science thinks that only a few parts of the whole are important (and therefore worth the cost of re-introducing). The analogy I have for this is a wardrobe: I am going to raid your wardrobe and take everything out of it, but I will only put back three items. Now, that's basically the same, isn't it? Of course not. So we must eat more whole foods. Fortified is better than non-fortified, but the whole food is far, far, superior.

Simple foods are better than those that are man-made and engineered. Tostitos® are made with corn, corn oil and salt, but to add the "touch of Lime," about a dozen ingredients have to be used. Lays® potato chips have sliced potato, oil, and salt. Baked Lays potato chips again require the addition of about a dozen more manufactured ingredients. Now, chips are not good for you and you shouldn't have them often and I only point this out to illustrate how a pretty simple recipe can be bastardized. I'm sorry, but we all need to start reading labels.

And I think it should go without saying, but please **Avoid Fast Food**, which is so processed, artificial, and unhealthy that to have it any more than once a month is too much. Even if they say it is low fat, or even "organic," don't be fooled into thinking it's healthy. Fast food is not healthy and it will make you fat, so it is best to avoid it completely.

However you change your diet or lifestyle, you should do so slowly and gently. If you try to change too much too fast, you will set yourself up to fail and you'll also shock your system. Detoxifying diets, liquid diets, fad diets, fasting diets, Atkins, South Beach, the chicken diet, etc., are neither balanced nor moderate. **The best way to get into balance is to live a little more in balance today than yesterday, and not to grossly overcompensate for yesterday's mistakes.** You did not get out of balance overnight, and food changes will not show improvement for a while. You do not need to detox, you just have to stop toxing. The toxins will work their way out of your system eventually as long as you stop replacing them. Do not make drastic changes; just try to do a little better this week than you did last week.

There are five main branches of Oriental Medicine: Acupuncture, Massage, Herbology, Dietary Therapy, and Exercise (tai-chi and Qi-gong). Dietary therapy is the best one to focus on because it is the most profound way we influence our bodies each and every day, whether we are aware of it or not. Most of my patients do not come to me in a state where a simple food change will be enough to correct their problem. But if we recognize that the diet, lifestyle and attitudes are at least partial causes of our disorders, then there is more we can do to help ourselves. Plus, if diet and lifestyle contributed to the development of a problem, then things will surely get worse if we do not change.

NOTE: For more in-depth information on Oriental Medicine, please see Chapter 18, where I elaborate on this topic.

Chapter Two

Grains

If carbohydrates were bad, most of Asia would not be thin. There is much research to show that a diet high in complex carbohydrates is the healthiest diet and one that is capable of reversing heart disease and diabetes. Most of our carbohydrates should come from grains, fruits and vegetables. Complex carbohydrates come from whole food products and break down appropriately in the body. Refined grains, such as white flour, are stripped of their nutrients and deliver sugar too fast to our bodies. Crackers, cookies, breads, and pastas (made with refined and/or bleached white flour) are not good sources of carbs.

Of the grains, **white rice is the best**. White rice has been much maligned in the public consciousness lately and has been lumped in with white bread, white sugar, and iceberg lettuce as a food devoid of value. Meanwhile, brown rice has been getting all the positive press. In general, I advocate eating whole foods with rice as somewhat of an exception.

Brown rice is white rice, with a thick coating around it. This shell is known as the germ layer, or bran, and this layer is what is "polished" off in making white rice. When analyzed in the lab, this germ layer is found to have some fiber and vitamins; but they have a poor bioavailability and most of it will just pass through us. Fiber is indigestible and just adds bulk to your stool. You can, and should, get all the vitamins and fiber you need from vegetables and fruits. Brown rice and white rice have roughly the same number of calories, but brown rice has more fat.

Eating the rice with this germ layer is a little like eating a walnut and not taking off the shell. Of course, nature had to put some nutrients into that coating to create it, but those nutrients are not very accessible to us. Our bodies will spend a great deal of time (largely unsuccessfully) trying to break through the covering and most of the material will eventually pass through us resulting in a loss of energy and a slowing of our metabolism. A little bit of brown rice can be helpful for certain types of constipation because the extra fiber helps bulk up the stool; but too much brown rice can actually exacerbate constipation by slowing the metabolism.

Brown rice was popularized with the macrobiotic movement and studies were carried out using brown rice as it is found in Japan, which is partially milled: that is to say that about 75% of this germ layer has already been removed. The brown rice that we get here in the United States is completely unshucked, so unless you are going to mill it yourself, brown rice will be a tall order for your body to digest.

The Chinese eat almost everything, including a lot of things that we would scoff (or even retch) at the mere thought of eating. When I was studying in China, I ate snake, pork kidneys, sea cucumbers and beef testicles, to name a few. So the fact that the Chinese go to the trouble to polish off the germ layer of brown rice indicates there must be a good reason: they found that it is easier to digest. If removing the germ layer of brown rice had led to a deficiency, the Chinese would have figured that out by now.

White rice is the most hypo-allergenic, easily assimilated, and energetically neutral of the grains. As I mentioned in the last chapter, all foods and herbs have properties – some things are warming or cooling, moistening or drying, activating or sedating, etc. White rice is completely neutral, so you could eat it all day, every day, and it would not throw off your internal energetic balance. It is true that it does have a high glycemic index, so persons with diabetes should exercise greater moderation and so white rice, like all things, should not be over-consumed.

White rice is also a very good first food to give to babies, being hypoallergenic and easy to digest and it has no gluten. After long illnesses and after traumatic events, patients in China are often given rice soup, called congees, to help with recovery. Normally, cooking rice calls for two cups of water to each cup of rice. To make a congee, use eight cups of water for each cup of rice and cook it for at least three to four hours over low heat. Congees can be served plain (translated bland), or they can be made sweet or savory. To sweeten it, you can add brown sugar, honey, raisins, bananas, etc., as you would with oatmeal. To make it savory, mince some meat, brown it and add some scallions, garlic, ginger and a pinch of salt.

So white rice is the best, but you shouldn't have it every day. All foods have things that are good and bad about them and **every food has something that nothing else can give you.** Another important principle of Asian food therapy is: **A good diet should be like a good stock portfolio – diversified**. If you have the same thing every day, or even every week, you are loaded up in one sector. This makes you more prone to the negatives of that sector, and at the same time, you are missing out on all the other good things happening in the market. So like a good portfolio, you should hedge your bets. All foods pull us in a particular direction and if you have just a little bit of different foods in your diet, nothing can pull you too far out of balance. Too much of any one food is not a good idea, and too little of any particular food is also not a good thing either. So you should include all the grains that are available in your diet: barley, millet, couscous, quinoa, flax, oats, rye, buckwheat, corn, job's tears, spelt, hemp seed, and sorghum. Even brown rice should be included in moderation. Actually, modern refining techniques are now much more effective than in the old days. In the past, white rice would have more of that germ layer left on it and that was good. For this reason, therefore, it is good to have some brown rice in your diet.

Not surprisingly, gluten intolerance is a growing problem, and it makes sense that too much of any one thing is not a good thing. For instance, we have been overdosed on wheat as it is used as filler for many processed foods such as crackers, cookies, and snack foods. And this same overdosing is also beginning to occur with soy, as soy lethicin is being injected into more processed foods. Thus the reason why whole foods are better is because you know exactly what is in them.

Therefore, a general rule with all foods is: **the more processed a food is, the more difficult it is to un-process**. Rice is popped out of its shell and steamed; wheat is popped out of its shell, then ground, mixed, heated, kneaded, leavened, and baked to make bread. This obviously takes a few more steps than rice, as does pasta. This is not to say that breads or pastas are bad, they are just a little more difficult for us to process and should represent a smaller proportion of our weekly intake. I have no idea how many steps are involved in making a Twinkie®, but I'm sure it's a great many! So Twinkies should really be kept at a minimum; and if you are trying to lose weight, you should avoid breads and pastas (and Twinkies) as much as possible.

The more robust your constitution is, the more you may be able to get away with eating processed foods. Some people can handle difficult-to-digest foods better than others, for a while. But remember, you either boost or injure your constitution every day with the food choices you make. Don't take good health for granted. Simple foods are simple to digest; and we want efficient digestion.

Chapter Three

Vegetables

The bulk of your diet should be vegetables and when compared with the Asian diet, our meals are unbalanced in America. We tend to eat a large protein, a small vegetable, and a small starch for our meals. Instead, we should be serving a large vegetable, a small protein, and a small starch. In fact, there is protein and starch in vegetables anyway, so you can eat all the vegetables you want and you should never go hungry.

Commercial over-farming has taxed the land of much of its nutrients and not all vegetables are created equal. Try to buy organically grown foods as often as you can. Local farms tend to use more sustainable methods and fewer chemicals than the big industrial farms, plus the vegetables are fresher and do not need to be preserved in transport. As a result, the foods have more nutrients and they contain a lot more life. Food that is full of life will give you life. Non-organic food is not bad for you; it is just not nearly as good for you. Pesticides and man-made fertilizers are very bad for you. Over the past 50 years, the USDA has noted a decline in the nutritional content of our produce, which should alarm us all. Could it be that we are eating more because our foods do not sufficiently nourish us?

We are also losing the diversity of vegetables in the pursuit of commercial farming profits. There are dozens of varieties of broccoli, but the agribusinesses only cultivate one. They are selecting and cultivating crops based on their yield, not on their quality or nutritional content. Genetic modification is altering our foods in ways we do not fully understand, and it is possible that we will lose the original foods as they are replaced by engineered variants. There is an excellent project called Seed Savers, which is trying to preserve seeds of all the un-altered produce in the world. Without intervention like this, it is possible that our only choices for produce in the future will be genetically modified ones. Please visit www.seedsavers.org and lend support to this important project.

Remember that you are constantly rebuilding your house and just as you would when rebuilding your home, you would naturally use the best materials available. And it is the same when you are rebuilding your body – you need high-quality material and this means organic. Organic, organic, organic. Better yet, grow your own vegetables (without pesticides or man-made fertilizers), and use heirloom seeds.

Cooked vegetables are better than raw. There are raw-food proponents out there who argue that, "Cooking a vegetable destroys all its nutrition." This is not true if that vegetable is cooked correctly. Lightly steaming or sautéing a vegetable does destroy about 10% of the nutrients, but the remaining 90% is then unlocked and available. **Everything cold and raw that you put in your stomach has to be heated and cooked internally by you.** This takes your body time and energy, and slows your metabolism. Calories, however, are a different concept than energy. The average Chinese person consumes 25-40% more calories per day than the average American. So it is not only the number of calories you eat, but how your body handles them. We need to get all the energy we can from our food so that we can then be active and burn up all the calories and eliminate the ones we don't need. As we get almost all of our energy from the food we eat, we don't want to spend too much energy processing this food. Otherwise it is like taking out $10 at an ATM and paying a $2 fee for doing so.

At one time there used to be some misinformation circulating about celery, which you may have heard that said celery was a 'negative food' because it costs more calories to process than it gives you, so you can eat it all day and you'll lose weight. Now, that would be great if it worked that way, but it doesn't. This will impair your digestion and slow your metabolism and is obviously inefficient. **What we want is efficient digestion.** We want our digestive tract to be like a filter – sending the good material to the tissues and the waste to the tissue paper. We don't want to expend too much time or energy having our bodies cooking that food. So we cook our food outside the body and lighten the load on our digestive tract, thus speeding up our metabolism in the process. **The less efficient our digestion is, the more food our bodies will ask for.**

In America, we tend to think that a salad is the healthiest thing we can eat. We all know someone who is trying to lose weight, who eats a big salad everyday, and yet is not losing weight. For one thing our salads can be incredibly bad for us with all the bacon, dressing, cheese, eggs, etc. that get piled on them sometimes. But even if the salad consists of just a plate of raw vegetables without dressing, that meal is too difficult to digest. Eating a small salad every now and then is fine, but a big salad every day is too much. The cell walls of plants are thick and are well defended, so cooking is a form of pre-digestion, which unlocks the nutrients.

Another way to pre-digest food is with fermentation. Asians pickle a lot of vegetables and eat them over the winter when fresh ones are not available. I wouldn't suggest eating pickled vegetables all the time, but they are good to add to your diet. In America, we pickle cucumber, pickles, beets, onions to name a few; but did you know that most vegetables can be pickled, including carrots, turnips, radish, peppers, tomatoes, cabbage, and many others? In the pickling process anti-microbial herbs such as mustard, garlic, cinnamon, and cloves are added to the solution to keep it from spoiling. Pickling preserves foods by creating an acidic environment in which harmful bacteria cannot grow but healthful microbes can. These microbes break down the food, creating natural pro-biotics, which also aids digestion.

Chinese Medicine and philosophy are all about the natural way. Sometimes my patients will say, "Isn't raw the natural state?" Yes, that is true, but it was not long after humans harnessed fire that they figured out how to use it to cook food, not just for meat but for vegetables as well. They noticed that the foods digested better when they were cooked and since then cooking has been a part of every recorded culture. In earlier days, people used to pay attention to how their bodies reacted to their diet and adjusted their eating accordingly. Sadly, nowadays we pay no attention to the ways different foods and different preparations affect us.

I imagine that some vegetables sitting out in the hot sun could be nearly cooked when they are plucked and eaten. So the natural state for a vegetable is from room temperature to hot; however, eating raw broccoli at 35 degrees Fahrenheit is un-natural. Refrigeration is great for preservation, but we should let the food warm up before we eat it. You can steam the vegetables ahead of time, keep them in the fridge, and then let them warm up to room temperature before eating. This will still be a lot easier on our digestions than eating them raw and cold.

While encouraging you to cook, I should clarify here that you usually don't want to overcook the vegetables. Overcooking vegetables can destroy most of the nutrition, so you don't want to kill them and make them all mushy. You want to cook vegetables long enough to bring them up to body temperature and soften them a little. Sometimes, after long illnesses or in times of weakness, you do want your food to be very well cooked. Soups and stews are very easy to digest and can be very nourishing, but most of your vegetables should only be slightly cooked.

Balance and moderation are the overriding principles. So please let me be clear: I am not recommending that you never have anything cold or raw. **You can and should have most foods in most forms.** However, to create balance, you should lean towards the cooked and warm foods primarily.

When I say you should have more vegetables, I do not mean just your three favorites. I read somewhere that the average American in a year eats between seven to eight different vegetables. God gave us a few more than that. **Every food has something that nothing else can give us.** No matter how much cauliflower you eat it will not equal broccoli; and there is no supplement that will equal cauliflower (more about this later). Don't take pride in having broccoli everyday, rather pride yourself on the wide variety of vegetables you consume.

Some estimates show that a full 60% of our calories come from four plants: wheat, soy, rice, and corn. Mostly these are not in their natural state, however, but in highly processed forms such as high-fructose corn syrup (a super sweetener) and soy lecithin (a filler). Eat natural foods and you will not be overdosed on these four.

In Asia, far more foods are included in their diets than we use in America. We all know that we can eat radishes, but did you know that we can also eat the radish tops? They are an excellent leafy green vegetable, as are dandelion greens, mustard greens, and turnip greens. Koreans make a jelly out of acorns; and the stems of a sweet potato can be marinated and taste delicious. Also don't forget about sea vegetables, such as seaweed and kelp, which are incredibly nutritious. There are many more available foods that we neglect when we confine our diets to the most tasty or easiest-to-prepare. Remember, we are not only feeding our tongues, so we need to diversify the portfolio and get more tastes and textures into the rotation.

Next time you are at the market, please take note of how many things they carry in the produce section that we **never** use. (There are still many items that I don't even know how to use.) Slowly try to expand your palette and every month, add one or two new foods. There are hundreds of recipe sites on the Internet that can give you suggestions on how to use these new foods. If you are feeling adventurous, check out the produce at the Asian markets and experiment with things like lotus root, Chinese cabbage, persimmon, and more.

Asian cooking tends to incorporate many different vegetables, and a typical Chinese stir-fry might contain over a dozen veggies. Koreans serve 5-30 pahn-chaans (little side dishes of different prepared vegetables and other foods) at most meals and eating a little of many foods makes sure you do not have too much of any one.

Eat local

There is a new trend in the health-conscious crowd called the locovores. Carnivores eat meat, herbivores eat plants, omnivores eat everything, and locovores only eat local food. I don't think you need to go overboard with this, but there is some sense to it. We have evolved in different parts of the world with different foods for good reason. It is not by coincidence that the parts of the world where a lot of spicy food is eaten tend to be by the equator. In equatorial regions, that spicy energy is needed to open the pores, causing sweating, and cooling the body down. Jalapenos do not grow in Canada as people don't need that energy there.

This is not to say that spicy peppers should never be eaten, but it is not good to eat a very tropical diet when not living in a tropical region.

My practice is in Chicago and I notice that many Indian immigrants have trouble because they want to keep eating the spicy curries and coriander of their native land. This spice suits the climate of South India, but it does not suit the midwestern climate. As a result, they can overheat themselves.

Another benefit of locally grown food is that it will be much fresher, and therefore more alive, when you eat it. We get our life-force from the life of the food we consume. Foods that are grown on the other side of the world can take weeks to be delivered; and they use carbon dioxide, wax, and food coloring to make it look fresh. No matter how it is preserved, the closer to freshly picked produce, the better it is. So be sure to check out your local farmer's market.

Our diets should consist mostly of local foods, slightly cooked. When changing to a new type of diet, people always need direction and ask many questions. In answer to questions such as whether it is better to eat more root vegetables or leafy ones, the answer is "Yes." And in response as to whether it is better to eat broccoli or asparagus, again I say "Yes." You should eat most foods-greens, reds, yellow, purples, roots, flowers, stems, leaves, and seeds, etc. If you do that, you have no choice but to eat moderately.

Chapter Four

Fruit

Fruit is different when compared to vegetables, but many people see them as basically interchangeable. They are on the same shelf of the food pyramid and therefore people see them as being the same and our only source of vitamins and minerals. However, their energies are really very different with the energy of fruit being much more sticky and dampening than that of vegetables.

Much of the Chinese understanding of the world began with rudimentary observation. First they developed hypotheses and then they tested them; and they discovered that there are many exceptions to every rule! But through this research they found that the energies of foods differ. For instance, if you squeeze an orange, the residual juice left on your hand is thick and sticky; but if you squeeze a piece of broccoli, it's mostly made up of water. **The way things are outside the body is how they will act inside the body.** The Chinese are very concerned with good circulation, therefore the Qi (energy), blood, food, fluids, thoughts, and emotions should all flow freely and sticky impairs free circulation.

Now to be clear, you should eat fruit, and you should have some every day, just not a ton of it. Have your vegetables in excess, fruit in moderation. The sticky-damp nature of fruits is more pronounced in tropical fruits for in the tropics, you need that energy as it is hot and you sweat. You do need to replace those fluids lost through sweating and you need to hold on to those fluids. A sticky, damp-natured food helps to retain fluids. I live in the Midwest and the fruits that grow here tend to be a little drier-apples, cherries etc. Even watermelon is not dry, but it is nowhere near as sticky as a pineapple or a mango. This is not to say that you can't ever have tropical fruits, but the majority of your fruit intake should come from those that are locally grown. And just like vegetables, you should have a wide variety and not eat the same fruit every day. It is impossible to be moderate when you always do the same thing. It is also easier to digest fruit that has been cooked, as it is not natural to ingest cold fruit; so you can bake an apple or make a fruit soup. Raw fruit eaten at room temperature is still much better for the body than fruit eaten straight out of the fridge.

Juice, by definition, is not moderate: it is a concentrate. Most of us would probably never sit down and eat six oranges, yet a large glass of orange juice may contain the equivalent of six oranges. I had a patient once who came in boasting that, thanks to his juicer he had a whole head of celery for his breakfast. When would anyone eat a whole head of celery? That is not moderate. The same principle applies to tomato sauce. Anyone who has cooked a homemade spaghetti sauce knows that you start with a pot full of tomatoes and simmer them down to 1/4 of the volume. Using this method, I am probably putting at least three or four tomatoes on my average plate of spaghetti. Again, that is not moderate (and remember that tomato is a fruit). So these days I try to eat a larger portion of vegetables and have a smaller side of pasta most of the time. This is not to say that you should never have juice or sauce, but when you do have it, recognize that you are having a concentrated food and practice even greater moderation: for instance, I usually water my juice down. By the way, if you want to drink juice, freshly squeezed is much better, as the longer a food (or juice) sits, the more it dies.

The juice rule also goes for protein shakes, breakfast shakes, and other concentrated meal-substitutes: they are never as good as the source food.

Western medicine suggests that you eat lots of fruits and vegetables. I recommend you have lots of vegetables – and fruits in moderation. The more tropical the region in which you live, the more fruit you can consume. But the majority of your intake should be vegetables, then grains, then a little of everything else.

Chapter Five

Proteins: Meat, Fish, Poultry, Tofu

Meat is rich and difficult to digest and most Americans consume far too much meat and that is not good. Excessive meat intake can cause all sorts of health problems ranging from obesity to hypertension, heart disease, to leukemia, Alzheimer's disease, and more. Meat increases hormone levels, resulting in earlier puberty, a higher risk of breast, prostate, and colorectal cancer, and sets the stage for a worse experience at menopause.

Cholesterol levels in America tend to be almost double those found in China and high cholesterol is associated with a higher intake of animal protein. Higher levels of cholesterol are also associated with a greater risk of heart disease, cancer and leukemia. Plants have no cholesterol and we do not need cholesterol in our diet.

Many people think that meat is the only source of protein. They further think that the only way to build muscle is with huge amounts of protein, which to them means meat (or supplements). However, we can get all the protein we need from plants and, in fact, Bill Pearl, who won the Mr. Universe contest four times, is a vegetarian. So you **can** build muscle without meat.

It is only recently that humans have had the luxury of eating meat with most meals. Before refrigeration was invented and became widespread, meat was an occasional food for most people. As it became more available, meat was seen as a sign of wealth. We need to correct this mindset. Now just because we are so wealthy as a nation and many can eat meat with every meal, it doesn't mean that it is a good thing.

In his book *The China Study,* Dr. T. Campbell describes the different causes of death as "diseases of poverty" and "diseases of affluence." The diseases of poverty include such ailments as malnutrition, parasites, and pneumonia, while the diseases of affluence include diseases such as diabetes, cancer, and heart disease. The increased meat intake that comes with affluence is probably the greatest factor in promoting these diseases. In addition to helping prevent such diseases, reducing meat intake can actually reverse heart disease and may also do the same for cancer. You can get all the protein you need from plants, especially beans, nuts, and peas.

So while most Americans eat too much meat, vegetarians do not consume any, which I believe is also not good. Remember **too much or too little of any one thing is not a good thing.** Chinese medicine recommends we have about two ounces of specifically mammal protein, twice a week. Fish is good and chicken is good, but we do need a little bit of mammal in our diet, the theory being that we, as mammals, are at a higher level of organization than plants, fish, or fowl and in order to keep ourselves functioning optimally at that higher level, we need a little bit of that raw material (mammal) in our diet. Most Americans greatly exceed this two-ounce, twice weekly allowance. I suggest that you think of meat as a condiment rather than as a main dish and you will do much better.

I give this information to all my patients and I have given it to large groups as well. I upset many vegetarians when I get to this point in the talk and so to all the veggies reading this, I am sorry. Many people think that vegetarianism is a healthy lifestyle, but in my opinion it is not. I think this is symptomatic of our extreme way of thinking: "If eating too much of something is bad, then to eat none of it must be good." Vegetarians almost have it right but they just eat a little too little mammal.

Vegetarians tend to be very committed to their diet and are proud of that commitment and I am sorry to have to challenge their mindset. A famous Chinese medical doctor, Miriam Lee, once wrote that "Vegetarianism is only appropriate for those whose main activity is meditation and whose lives are lived in the shelter of a temple." (*Insights of a Senior Acupuncturist*, page 52). Those of us with a more active lifestyle need a little more of an active food source.

One of the things that we get from red meat (and which doesn't sound appealing) is blood. As I explain in Chapter 18 about Oriental Medicine, blood nourishes the tissues, but it also calms the spirit. Long-term vegetarians tend to develop a condition called blood deficiency and they tend to become pale, emaciated, sickly, have thinner hair and brittle nails, and can be prone to anxiety and insomnia; they are also less resistant to disease. Without sufficient blood, the menses can be affected and fertility impaired. It is well-known in Oriental Medicine that vegetarian women have a harder time becoming pregnant.

In the United States most of us eat far too much meat. Then, when we change our diet and give up eating meat, we start to feel better: our bowels work better, we feel lighter and more energetic, and we wonder why we didn't do this years ago. However, as the years go by, and we have worked off the excess meat, we begin to develop these blood deficiencies, which most people never attribute to the vegetarianism. "I gave up meat 10 years ago, why should I just be having this problem now?" they ask. It is because they had a large imbalance to work off, and because food changes take a long time to play out.

As for the humanitarian argument, I believe that **God loves carrots too**. Every living thing has a life-force and works to stay alive and reproduce. That carrot would prefer to continue to live to a ripe old age in the ground rather than being plucked from its home and diced into my salad. For anything to live and grow, something must be sacrificed. Everything eats something. It is not possible to "do no harm" and stay alive and healthy, so that is not the goal. The goal is to be mindful and thankful for everything that had to die to support our lives. Most of us do not give the appropriate thought or thanks for the things that are sacrificed to keep us alive. This is also a reason why we should not waste food and the simple act of saying grace before meals can help to remind us that we are fortunate to have this fuel so we can continue our lives.

Buddhism is widespread in Asia; and one of the main tenets of Buddhism is to have compassion for all creatures great and small. Everything and everybody has energy and that energy can be imprinted into the physical being. To treat our livestock cruelly damages their energy (and our karma), and although ultimately our animals may end by being slaughtered to feed humans, those lives should be free and full. Our animals should be free of hormones and antibiotics, able to roam the land and interact with other animals, and be afforded a natural diet. Nature shows us when we are doing things wrong. For instance, many farmers use antibiotics because the cattle are housed in overcrowded conditions, and mad cow disease came from feeding the cows an unnatural diet (where the food included ground up cattle by-products). So if we treat the animals more naturally and humanely, they will be far less prone to disease and won't therefore need medications.

In order to maintain a balanced diet, we should not always eat the same cuts of meat from the same animals either. For most of us, the only form of meat we have is muscle from cows, pigs, fish, or chickens. It is only recently in the Western world that we have discarded so much of the animal and only consumed the muscle, whereas in most traditional cultures, every edible part of an animal is consumed: muscle, organs, glands, tripe, and even brains. The functions and makeup of the organs and glands are very different from that of the muscles, so we are missing out by not incorporating these energies into our diet. Liver is well known to be one of the healthiest meats we can eat, but most of us never eat it; we should include it in our diets at least once in a while.

Just as it is important for us to have a wide variety of foods, our animals have that same need. Cattle that are fed only grain or corn are lacking the diversity that they naturally consume when they free-range where they will eat grass, dandelions, grains, and a host of other foods. By limiting their diet, we impair the nutritional value of the meat. Our animals should be allowed to have a natural diet.

The Jewish tradition (Kosher) and the Middle eastern tradition (Halal) both dictate that the animal must be killed in a humane way. These cultures recognize that this affects the energy of the meat; and we know that the food we eat affects our energy. I think this makes sense, for if an animal is scared, it will release the fear hormones and those hormones will be present in that meat. Do you really want to put more fear hormones into your body? Of course not, but this concern for the way an animal dies does not go far enough. A humane killing will not undo a life of deprivation and mistreatment and it is not enough to end their lives humanely: we must allow them to live their lives humanely as well.

The following are suggestions regarding other types of meat.

Lunchmeat
Buy freshly sliced meat from the deli as pre-packaged lunchmeat is processed and includes preservatives. (This is also true for frozen chicken breasts). Buy fresh and freeze them yourself, although it is always best to eat fresh, unfrozen food.

Fish
Some people do not eat meat on ethical grounds, but will eat fish. When the Christians came to Tibet and encouraged the people there to eat fish (the food of Jesus) instead of yaks, they disagreed. "Why should we sacrifice 100 souls to feed the village when we can sacrifice just one?" This is not to say that we should only eat bigger animals, we should eat a variety of foods. But, frankly, I don't understand those who object to the killing of a cow and not to the killing of a fish. Farmed fish are usually overcrowded and diseased and like cattle, fish should be farmed in a humane way. Eating an excessive amount of fish can give us too much mercury, which can cause neurological problems among other health issues. So fish, like most foods, should be eaten in moderation.

It is a huge tragedy and disgrace that we have polluted our water to the point where we cannot safely eat the fish caught from large bodies of water such as Lake Michigan, where I live. This natural resource should be able to feed all the communities that surround it. Currently it is recommended that people consume no more than one serving of fish per month from Lake Michigan, because the water (and therefore the fish) is so polluted. For this reason alone, we must stop dumping chemicals into our water supply and lakes.

A note on sushi
I recommend limiting raw food as part of The Asian Diet and people often ask about sushi. For one thing, Japanese people do not eat sushi as often as we think. They usually eat stir-fried vegetables, rice, and noodle dishes. Sushi in Japan is

served with warm rice, miso soup, and hot tea and these additions help warm up the raw fish in the stomach. And, by the way, pickled ginger and wasabi are served with sushi because they are both antimicrobial and antibacterial, and not just added for taste.

Chicken and Poultry

Chicken and other poultry are fine and desirable in moderation as long as they are not always fried or drenched in sauce or oil. White meat is not better than dark, so rotate the poultry parts, and don't only eat breasts and wings. As with the larger animals, you want to eat free-range, hormone-free, antibiotic-free, happy chickens that are sacrificed in a humane manner.

Eggs

Eating eggs is natural: for instance, many species feed themselves on the eggs of other species. I also find it amusing when people will eat eggs but not chickens: eggs are just chicken futures. **Egg whites are not better than egg yolks.** This is another example of humans trying to separate that which nature has combined. Together they are both Yin and Yang. Egg whites are very sticky, and can be used to make glue and adhesives. Once again, it's good to remember that the way foods are outside the body is how they act inside the body and glue is not helpful to our vital circulation. Neither egg yolks nor whites are particularly good for us, so they should be taken in moderation and only eaten maybe once or twice per week.

Tofu

Many people, when they give up meat, tend to overdo the soy. They will have a soy burger with soy cheese; wash it down with soy milk, with edamame on the side. Tofu is great in moderation and is also a useful way to help cut your meat intake. My wife and I make stir-fries pretty regularly. We used to add two chicken breasts into our stir-fry; now we add just one breast plus a package of tofu. Tofu is the great wild card of the culinary world, as it will adopt the flavors with which you are cooking: cooked with chicken, it tastes like chicken; and cooked with beef, it tastes like beef. I prefer the firm texture tofu (it feels more like meat), but now that I'm used to it, I can enjoy the soft tofu as well. As always, organic and fresh is best.

Tempeh, Seitan, and other "meat substitutes"

I don't like the term "meat substitute." It is like calling lettuce a "cabbage substitute." They are their own foods and have good things to offer. Tempeh is a great source of protein. There is no problem with eating these "substitutes", but as with most things, don't overdo them. Seitan, by the way, is made from wheat gluten and is therefore not appropriate for those with gluten intolerance.

Nuts

Enjoy your nuts, but don't go nuts. They are great sources of fiber and protein and can be eaten toasted or roasted. However, if you grind the nuts up and make a concentrate, and dissolve this concentrate into oil (as in peanut butter) you negate the positives that nuts give you. So let me be clear: **nuts are good; nut butters are not as good,** as they are sticky and heavy. Again, the way things are outside the body is how they will act inside the body.

Beans

Beans are fabulous, so have as many as you want, but don't always eat the same ones.

As with most suggestions in this book, I recommend you adjust your meat intake gradually. If you are used to having meat with 14 meals a week, try to cut down to 12, then 10, then eventually two meals that include meat. If, however, you are at the other end of the spectrum and have not eaten meat in a long time, please re-introduce it slowly. At first, it will be hard to digest and we don't want to make this transition unpleasant, so start with one small bite and then wait a few days before eating any more. Beef-based soups can also be a good way to begin to re-introduce meat into your diet.

Food changes take a long time take effect, so don't expect drastic and fast improvements, this is slow and gentle change. However, if you do not change your eating habits, your nose dive will continue, you will get further out of balance, and it will take longer to undo the damage.

Chapter Six

Soups

Many Asian cultures have soup with most meals and they say the ideal rule for eating a balanced meal is that your stomach should be half full of food and a quarter full of fluids, thus you don't fill your stomach to capacity at each meal. The fluids include soups, but not cream-based soups (unless you are trying to put on weight).

Soups are nourishing and very easy to digest, especially if you use a bone in the cooking, as bones are very nutritious. The warm fluid facilitates digestion in the stomach and according to one concept in Chinese culture the contents of our stomach should create a 100-degree soup (37°C). Making soup can seem time consuming, but once made, you can eat it for several days. There are dozens of different soups, do not just stick with your three favorites. If you have to buy prepared soup, choose one in a box rather than in a can as cans are liable to leach metals into the food. Unfortunately, most packaged soups are overloaded with sodium and preservatives. Also do not microwave soup (more about the dangers of microwaving later).

Soups are a good way to lose weight as it fills up your stomach with easy-to-digest fluid. Four ounces of meat is not much when served as a steak, but diced into a soup it goes a long way.

In particular:

Beef soup is good for anemia and weakness.

Chicken soup is good for fatigue, chronic fatigue, and fibromyalgia.

Mung bean soup is good for inflammation of the internal organs (hepatitis, pancreatitis, appendicitis, etc).

Mushroom soup nourishes the liver (learn about the function of the liver in Chapter 18).

Clam soup treats hypertension.

Bone marrow soup is called "longevity soup" and utilizes the crushed bones of chicken and pork legs.

Using a slow cooker or crock-pot makes fixing soups easy, and keeps it warm and on-hand, just like the rice-cooker (for more about a rice-cooker, see Chapter 21). The crock-pot used to be a staple in American cooking but is now almost never seen. I suggest you buy one and start using it.

Chapter Seven

Dairy

I have said earlier that you should eat a little of most foods; however, you don't ever need dairy. Well, I wouldn't say this to everybody, but I can tell you since you are old enough to be reading this book. Infants do need dairy, but that should be specifically mother's milk. Humans are the only mammals that drink milk after infancy. **Dairy is really intended for infants.** Once we have our teeth, we are ready for real food and this is why the breasts usually stop lactating when the child is about 18-24 months. By that age we don't need it anymore. We are also the only animal that drinks the milk of another animal. Even if our cows were hormone free, antibiotic-free, free-range, and very happy cows, it is still not the way that we were designed to get our nutrition. If in the unlikely event that a choice has to be made between starving and dairy, then of course dairy would be important and should be utilized. But if you have other options, stick with those.

The Dairy Boards of America have spent a lot of money and done a fantastic job of "educating" us about the need for milk and I am amazed at how effectively they have done this. Their campaigns begin in grade schools where milk is the only beverage option and they poster the walls in the schools spreading "Milk is Healthy" propaganda. They also pay beloved celebrities to promote their products and have even managed to obtain the responsibility of educating future doctors in medical schools by providing the educational materials. If the dairy industry is educating doctors, do you think they will ever let them know that there are health problems associated with consuming milk? The bedfellows of the food industry are powerful and are willing to sacrifice public health in the pursuit of profits.

These state and national councils sound like government agencies, but they are professional trade groups, made up of the people who produce and distribute milk. They have a vested interest in promoting the concept that milk is good for us, in the same way the Orange Juice Growers' Associations paid for the commercials teaching us how good orange juice is for us. And it's guys like me who will tell you how good acupuncture is! We have a vested interest in promoting our products and services and are therefore a questionable source. The dairy commercials imply that if we don't have our three servings a day, our bones will go brittle and break. I would like to ask the dairy councils, "Why do horses have strong bones?" They don't eat yogurt – they eat green leaves. **Green leafy vegetables are the best source of calcium.**

I believe (as I have mentioned above) that humans are the only animals that drink milk after infancy, but not all humans do so, it is primarily Europeans and their descendants. They don't use milk in Africa or Asia and there is no higher incidence of osteoporosis in Asia than in America. In fact, there are fewer hip fractures (the number one complication of osteoporosis) in Asia. This is often attributed to the bone-promoting value of green tea, which Asians drink all the time.

So, clearly, milk is not the only way to get strong bones; in fact, some experts believe that dairy impairs bone health. Europeans and Americans eat the most dairy products and actually have the weakest bones. At the end of this book, I list some tips for promoting bone health, and reducing dairy is one of the suggestions because the protein content of milk is very acidic and requires the body to pull calcium out of the bones to neutralize it.

Breast milk is best for developing infants as the mother is the immune system for the baby and she can make the antibodies and pass them to the baby. Substituting cow's milk cannot fulfill this important function. In addition, I believe that the early introduction of cow's milk increases the risk of the child developing type-one (juvenile) diabetes.

(If there is insufficient lactation, you may substitute a wet-nurse, organic goat's milk, soy milk, nut milks, and sprout milks. In this case, it will be helpful to juice green vegetables and also feed that to the baby. The juice can be mixed with the milks or fed separately).

Phlegm

Dairy is a food that turns to substance in the body. In an infant, that is exactly what we need, as babies need to make a lot of substance in a hurry. The internal fire of an infant is strong enough that it can transform this highly nutritive food into usable tissues. Beyond this time, it is over-nourishing the body and impairing the child's digestive system (possibly for life). The substance that dairy turns to in an adult body is phlegm.

Phlegm can manifest in many ways: it can lodge between the skin and the muscles as fat; it can stick in the lungs and cause respiratory problems like asthma and chronic obstructive pulmonary disorder; it can go to the throat causing a post-nasal drip; and it can occlude the sinuses causing sinus infections, sinusitis and rhinitis (many of my patients have been able to get off the roller coaster of sinus infection-antibiotics-sinus infection by cutting out dairy). It can also cause a mental fog and contribute to forgetfulness, dementia, and Alzheimer's disease; and in addition, it can also congeal to form cysts, fibroids and tumors. The Chinese understand cancer and these other abnormal growths basically as phlegm-balls, and they have noticed more growths in populations that consumed dairy. So they spread the word and now more people know to avoid it. In his book *The China Study*, Dr. Campbell convincingly shows how milk protein causes cancer and how eliminating it can stop its progression. He also points out that dairy products promote heart disease, and auto-immune diseases such as multiple sclerosis, lupus, rheumatoid arthritis, and more.

All dairy products are not created equal; for instance, skim milk is the most watery and lightest form of dairy, while cream is much heavier and thicker and cheese is the heaviest, densest and stickiest dairy product. Again, remember, the way things are outside the body is how they will act in the body. So if you want to be heavy and dense, eat a lot of cheese. Ice cream is the trifecta of cold and sticky and dairy and is one of the hardest things for your body to digest and will give you the least benefit. This is not to say that you can never eat ice cream, for nothing is so good that it should be taken all the time, and very few things are so bad that they need to be avoided like the plague. I tell my patients that they should try to get most foods into their diet, but they don't need to try with dairy. Most adults are intolerant to lactose, so what does this tell you? There is a product on the market called Lactaid®, which can be taken in order that we can continue to drink something that our bodies are clearly rejecting. I suggest, therefore, that you listen to your body and respect its wishes.

Yogurt is a somewhat different story. It has probiotics in it that help digest the dairy and also helps digest everything else in your stomach. Yogurt is the least damaging form of dairy, but should still only be taken in moderation.

The grocers of America have confused most Americans. Eggs are not dairy, even though they are in the same case at the market; dairy comes from cows, eggs come from chickens. Eggs are a natural food and, again, should be consumed in moderation; however, the eggs should come from humanely treated chickens that have free range and have no drugs added to their feed.

Bone health

Although this book does not endeavor to be a research paper with everything footnoted, please refer to Dr. HingHau Tsang's suggestions for bone health which I thought were worth including and which can be found in the Supplemental Information section at the end of this book. You can also find more information at: http://tsangenterprise.com/news122.htm

Chapter Eight

Beverages

Your first and most important fluid intake should be water and the next most important should be green tea. All other fluids should only be drunk in moderation.

Water is essential for proper functioning of the body and how much water a person needs really depends on many variables, such as: size, fitness, climate, weather, what foods you have been eating, digestive state (diarrhea can dehydrate you), bladder activity, etc. Doctors recommend eight glasses a day for everyone. I have never understood how one set amount of water can apply all of us. For instance, how can a 250-pound man working hard labor in the summer sun of the Colorado mountains have the same hydration needs as a 90-pound, inactive, elderly person living with a humidifier in Maine? For most of us, our bodies tell us when we need water and I think you should just drink when you are thirsty.

A small number of people never seem to feel thirsty and therefore do not drink enough fluid. If this is the case with you, you can use your urine as a gauge and it should be a pale yellow color; if it is dark yellow or orange, you need more water. We need to maintain an aqueous environment in our bodies. The theory is that all cells evolved in the sea; then they joined up: "You be the lung, I'll be the liver, let's find a leg and crawl our way out of here." In order to maintain our cells working without the ocean environment, we need to carry that environment with us; so if we do not have enough water, it is like boiling a soup too long – it gets too thick and concentrated.

Use only spring or filtered water

Most municipal water supplies use chemicals, some of which are added intentionally and some just wind up tainting the supply through pollution and inappropriate disposal methods. For instance, medications are often found in municipal water supplies because people flush their unused pills down the toilet. I worry enough about taking prescription drugs that have been prescribed for me, and worry even more about taking medicines of which I am unaware. In addition to the unwanted chemicals in our water, many municipalities actually add some intentionally, such as chlorine and fluoride among others. Chlorine is a poisonous gas and can combine with other elements in the water to form carcinogenic compounds. Fluoride in the water really does not help our teeth or bones, as it is not in the right form. Fluoride is found in certain plants and, from plant sources (like green tea), the fluoride seems to be effective and safe. Fluoride added to the water supply is man-made and is a byproduct of industrial manufacturing aluminum or fertilizer; in this form it can cause cancer, weaken bones, and impair fertility. In my view, it should be regarded as a hazardous material and disposed of properly, not fed to the unknowing public.

Think about how many products you consume that are made with fluoridated water: soups, juices, beer, wine, baby formula, bread, cakes, even processed cereals are made with municipal water. So unless it has gone through a reverse-osmosis filter, it probably contains fluoride. We can tolerate most things in moderation, but fluoride is now in so many products that we have all over-dosed on it. For this reason, spring water is best. The only way to get fluoride out of the water is through reverse-osmosis, which is costly and wasteful, plus it robs the water of its trace minerals. So the best thing would be if our governments just stopped adding it to everyone's water. To all the mayors and governors reading this, please stop fluoridating the public's water supply. Thank you.

And please do not use a new, plastic water bottle each time you want to take a drink. The environmental impact is ridiculous and, in addition, toxic dioxins can leech out of those bottles, into the water, and then build up in us. To learn about the frightening dangers of dioxins, read *Our Stolen Future* by Theo Colborn, Dianne Numanoski, and John Peter Meyers. Please use and re-use either glass or stainless steel containers for your water.

Soft drinks are aptly named because they will make you soft, as not only will the high doses of sugar contribute to your fat, but also the carbonation actually robs your bones of calcium. In addition, soft drinks contain numerous artificial chemicals. One of my general rules when checking labels is: was an ingredient in my grandmother's cabinet? If so, then it is probably OK. But if I have no idea what an ingredient is or where it came from, I find it is usually suspect. Next time you see one, take a look at the ingredients in Diet Coke®. I believe that if this drink were a drug, then it would be banned by the FDA (assuming the FDA was really working on behalf of public safety). If you really would like a cola now and then, that's fine, but you should get a REAL cola. Whole Foods and other health-food stores carry brands that only use carbonated filtered water, pure cane sugar, cola beans, and sea salt. I wouldn't drink them too often because they are sweet (sticky) and most often served very cold. Natural root beer and lemon-lime drinks are OK too, but make sure they do not contain synthetic sweeteners.

Coffee is a fine occasional drink

I know a lot of people are attached to their morning coffee (and beyond), so I like to start out with a positive. It is, however, a lousy everyday drink. For one thing, it is terribly addictive. Many of my patients report that they drink coffee everyday because they HAVE to, as they would either experience a terrible withdrawal headache, or they would be unable to function. I had a suite mate in college who used to wake me up every morning with a cup of freshly brewed coffee and this was great. But then he went home for a week, leaving his coffee maker in his locked room. I missed all my morning classes that week because I just could not drag myself out of bed. It occurred to me then that I had become addicted to coffee and I made the decision that I did not want to continue my dependence on it.

The energy of coffee is unbalanced: it has a frenetic energy, and the more you put in your body, the more unbalanced and frenetic your energy will become. Over-exposure to coffee can make people anxious, irritable, and impair attention and sleep and, as it contains a high dose of caffeine, it can cause myriad health problems. You only have to Google "dangers of coffee" and you can see all the things it does. Plus, the boost that coffee gives you has too sharp an onset and too sharp a crash. The energy you get is similar to using a credit card – you have to pay back more than you received. Coffee also disrupts your body's ability to regulate your own alertness. However, it is not pure evil, and is fine if used in moderation.

Green tea is the greatest beverage in the world

It prevents heart disease, vascular disease, cancer, cavities; it increases metabolism, decreases appetite, regulates blood sugar and blood pressure, lowers cholesterol, reduces pain, improves mood, and may even prevent chromosomal damage in the eggs and sperm. The more I learn about this tea plant, the more I am convinced that it came either directly from God, or from aliens! It is so good for so much and often in an unusual way. It is the only plant of which I am aware that stimulates both the sympathetic nervous system (a.k.a. the fight or flight response) with caffeine, but also stimulates the parasympathetic nervous system (the calm and relax response) with the compound L-Theanine. So it is a balanced substance: it wakes you up and calms you down, Yin and Yang. Caffeine from all sources impairs bone health, except for green tea, which improves bone density. Caffeine from all sources impairs fertility, except when in green tea, which has been shown to improve fertility. At my office, we see a lot of women who are trying to get pregnant and have read that they should avoid all caffeine. I like to point out to them that, if green tea impaired fertility, China would not have grown to over a billion people. Apparently there is something in green tea that neutralizes the negative effects of caffeine in addition to all the good things it gives us.

You should have at least one cup of regular green tea every day. I tell my patients: "If you smoke, the best thing you can do for your health is to quit smoking. If you do not smoke, the best thing you can do is to have one cup of regular green tea a day." Quitting smoking and drinking green tea are on the same order of magnitude in terms of their respective health benefits.

Some tea manufacturers use chemical processes to decaffeinate their tea so I do not recommend you buy decaffeinated green tea. In its regular form, it has enough caffeine to stave off the coffee headache, but not so much as to make you jittery. Sources vary in their measurements of caffeine, but your average cup of coffee has about 140 mg of caffeine; green tea has about 35 mg, and 90% of the caffeine is released in the first minute of brewing. So if you are really trying to minimize your caffeine intake, you can brew the leaves or tea bag for a minute, pour out the water and then brew it again. The second brew has only 3.5 mg of caffeine, about the same as in three Hershey®'s kisses. Most people should be fine with 35 mg of caffeine and will not need to discard the first brew.

The worst green tea is still better than the best coffee. Tea is sacred in China and is usually grown without using any pesticides or artificial chemical fertilizers. (This is usually not the case with coffee, which is regarded solely as a cash crop.) In China, they take their tea seriously. I am partial to the gunpowder tea or pearled tea, where the leaves are rolled (usually by hand) into tight little balls. This minimizes the surface area and therefore prevents the evaporation of the essential oils. Regular tea bags hold little, desiccated pieces of tea leaves, making for a huge surface area and greater evaporation, so I think the whole leaf is better and the rolled whole leaf is the best. Japanese tea is powdered and you can't have any greater surface area than that. Traditionally this method was quite appropriate, because the tea leaves were freshly ground right at the time they were making the tea. But again, the worst green tea is still better for you than the best coffee.

So what kind of tea should you buy? Whatever flavor you like. Most Americans are not turned on to green tea because they have never tasted a good one. When I was younger I had tea now and then and it tasted OK, but I was never really impressed with it and it made no sense to me that Britain would sail half way around the world to buy it. Finally, I tried a good tea. The analogy I use is tea and beer: all my life I had been drinking Schlitz®; and I couldn't understand what all the fuss was about beer, which I felt was a mediocre product at best. Then I tried a Samuel Adams® beer and I thought, "So that's what all the fuss is about." A good tea is like drinking a Sam Adams beer. Since then, I have become much more aware of the differences in tea quality and I am amazed at how prevalent Schlitz-quality tea is. Be assured, you do not need to spend exorbitant amounts of money on tea, as long as you find one that you like, any one will do.

People in some parts of the world like to drink black tea. The difference between green tea and black tea is the same as the difference between green bananas and black bananas: black bananas have more flavor, but they are dead. Black tea has twice the caffeine and one-tenth the health benefits and adding sugar and milk just gives even less health benefits. A little black tea now and then is fine, especially in the winter, but your staple should be green tea. White tea is also good and all herbal teas are fine in moderation.

One of the reasons that Asians tend to be thin is that they drink green tea with every meal. The tea helps to dissolve fat, which, as we have learned, is hard to digest. Lipitor® and other statin drugs keep cholesterol levels down by blocking its absorption in the liver. Green tea can dissolve cholesterol in the stomach, before it even enters the blood stream.

In addition, green tea is warm and warm fluids facilitate the process of digestion, while cold fluids impede it. The enzymes in the stomach work in a limited temperature range. If you cool the stomach below a certain threshold, you essentially turn off your digestion. Of course it doesn't stay turned off for very long – just long enough for the body to warm up the environment, but forcing the body to have to do this is counter-productive. We want to be able to process our food efficiently and send it on its way. Americans have ice-cold drinks with every meal and look at the shape of the average American. Keep your digestion moving and don't make things harder than they have to be. Fluids at body temperature are best and at room temperature are good, but ice-cold are the worst. Of course, the best guide is moderation and it is OK to have that cold lemonade on a nice summer day or sip a chilled white wine with your dinner once in a while.

Where did we get this obsession over ice-cold drinks? Historically, it was a show of wealth to be able to modify the temperature of foods and drinks. Nowadays, as refrigeration is widespread, restaurant owners have perpetuated the habit of adding ice to liquids; they like it because they can fill your glass three quarters full with ice (which is cheap) and then only have to give you a quarter of the product. It saves them a lot of money and robs you of that for which you have paid.

I have already covered fruit drinks and juices in Chapter 4. To repeat, fruit juices are concentrates and violate the moderation principle and should be taken only in moderation. I usually water juice down and don't drink it very often.

Alcohol has a drying and sedating effect, and overuse can lead the body to produce phlegm. So again, you don't want to put too much alcohol into your body either; and if you have a problem controlling your drinking, or controlling your behavior when you have been drinking, please do us all a favor and abstain. Alcohol has been used medicinally for millennia and red wine has some real health benefits; and, like everything else, it is OK in moderation. If you can't keep it in moderation, too little is better than too much.

Energy drinks contain too many concentrates to be moderate in any way, so stay away from them. Gatorade® and other sport drinks are loaded with electrolytes that are needed if you are exerting yourself for an extended period of time. They can be thought of as a medication, but not as a beverage. I do wish that Gatorade® would stop using high fructose corn syrup in their product.

Chapter Nine

Sugar Substitutes

Sweetening is a multi-billion dollar industry; money and politics have played shady roles in bringing these products to the market, and now they are everywhere. There are, however, a few ways to sweeten things naturally and they are: pure cane sugar (a.k.a. raw sugar), beet sugar, honey, stevia, agave nectar, maple syrup, molasses, rapidura, brown rice syrup, barley malt syrup, sucanat, turbinado sugar, date sugar, and fruit juice. All of these are fine and should be used in moderation.

Refined sugar is better than sugar substitutes, but it is still not good for you. Raw sugar actually has some nutrients and it contains a compound that protects the teeth. We could eat pure cane sugar all day and get no cavities. Refining the sugar is similar to refining grains in that the process strips away all the healthful components and only leaves us the sweetness. I think this should go without saying, but **Candy is bad**. Moderation here means less than one piece every few days, and optimally less than one to two pieces a month. You don't ever need it.

Most of the foods we eat have at least some sweetness to them. We have become desensitized to this because we eat so much concentrated sugar and sweets all the time. Eating ever sweeter and sweeter foods just takes us further away from being able to enjoy the inherent sweetness to be found in natural foods. It can be likened to looking directly into a spotlight for 20 minutes and then trying to appreciate candlelight. If we take a break from the artificially super-sweet products, we can regain the appreciation of the flavors of natural foods.

Too much sweet flavor, regardless of its source, engenders dampness and phlegm in the body and taxes the digestion. But **artificial sweeteners are much worse for us than sugar**. We have evolved eating sugar and our DNA has worked with glucose for thousands of years, never high fructose corn syrup, aspartame, Splenda, etc. These are unnatural products and I believe they are contributing to the rise of diabetes in this country. A pancreas knows how to handle glucose, but it doesn't know what to do with these new substances, and it is my belief that they disturb our insulin production. But there is big money in selling us sweeteners and we keep buying them.

High Fructose Corn Syrup (HFCS)

This is the cheapest way to get sweetness into your food products; and it has become ubiquitous; it is found in everything from candy and soda, to bread, yogurt, pizza, crackers, ketchup, and much more. Remember, too much of any one thing is not a good thing. Having HFCS in so many foods means that we are being overdosed on corn and fructose, which comes from corn that is genetically modified to increase its sweetness, and prepared with genetically modified enzymes. Plus, every individual cell in our bodies metabolizes glucose, but fructose is only processed in the liver, putting an additional strain on that organ.

HFCS is banned in Europe and Canada but the FDA in the USA claims that HFCS is natural. Can someone please show me the high-fructose corn plant that it comes from? It is not natural, it is man-made. This is another instance where special interest groups have compromised the government agencies that are supposed to be protecting us.

Aspartame (a.k.a. Nutrasweet®, Equal®)

Aspartame is what goes into Diet Coke®, Diet Pepsi®, and just about everything else that is sweet and diet. It is 180 times as sweet as sugar and many people believe they are helping their bodies by using this instead of sugar, but unfortunately they are quite wrong. Recent studies have shown that people using this sugar substitute experience an increased appetite! The use of diet sodas is associated with weight gain, not weight loss. Why then would you use this sweetener if you were trying to lose weight?

The fact that Aspartame® has no calories just means that our bodies cannot break it down. So even though it passes through the body it still has an impact; as this chemical makes it way through our bodies, it interacts with many other types of cells and structures.

There were many objections from the scientific community when Aspartame® was seeking approval from the FDA and subsequently, the FDA has received more complaints about this product than any other substance. Aspartame breaks down into formaldehyde in the body (a known carcinogen) and is associated with headaches/migraines, brain tumors, brain lesions, memory loss, arthritis, hypertension, abdominal pain, and lymphomas. But there was enough profit to be made that Donald Rumsfeld (then Chairman of Searle, the company holding the patent on Aspartame®) was able to get it approved. The FDA voted to ban the substance, but this vote was overturned through what I believe to have been some very shady politics: it was just too profitable and now Aspartame® is in over 5000 food products in the US. I know some people who often drink three or more diet sodas a day and think that they are better for them than regular sodas. However, I believe that micro dose by micro dose, these people are poisoning themselves. So please stay away from drinks containing this sweetener.

Another sweetener, Equal®, also contains aspartame, plus an additional ingredient distinguishing it from Nutrasweet®. This ingredient is phenylalanine, which can cause seizures at high doses.

Sucralose (Splenda®)

Sucralose is found in over 3,500 food products in the US and the makers, Johnson and Johnson, claimed that it is made of sugar; however, they are now being sued because that is not true. Sucralose has chlorine in it and while some other foods have naturally occurring chlorine, this is OK because they also contain additional compounds to neutralize its effects; but man-made chlorine is extremely toxic and can kill. Unlike aspartame, all sucralose does not travel through the body: about 15-27% of ingested sucralose is absorbed. How it behaves once absorbed is not yet understood, but anecdotal reports associate sucralose with headaches, urinary problems, fatigue, digestive disorders, and other ailments.

Saccharine (Sweet 'n' low®)

This was the first of the artificial sweeteners to bypass public safety and there has been opposition to this product for over 100 years. It is made from anthranilic acid, nitrous acid, sulfur dioxide, chlorine, and ammonia (obviously you would never eat any of these things if you had a choice). Even though saccharine has long been suspected to cause cancer, nevertheless it is still on the market.

A general rule is: **If God makes it, it's probably OK. If it is made by man, it is suspect.** (This does not apply to toadstools, arsenic, mercury, and other known, natural poisons). **Natural sweeteners are always better than the artificial ones.**

People with diabetes often feel they have no choice but to ingest these sugar substitutes. However, if you correct your diet, you can stabilize your blood sugar and be better able to tolerate the occasional encounter with sugar. Natural sugars are not so bad and by adopting a more plant-based, whole foods diet you can reduce or eliminate the need for diabetic medication. Monitor your sugars and, when and if appropriate, discuss tapering your medication with your physician. But DO NOT alter your medication based on information in this book.

Chapter Ten

Supplements

Supplements are a billion-dollar industry and, in my view, supplements can be great and they can be exactly what you need, **provided they are exactly what you need today**. Many people have this notion that supplements can only be good and cannot be bad for you. Of course, nothing is so one sided: too much or too little of anything can be equally out of balance. **You should get most of your nutrition from your food.** This is how we have evolved.

Many people seem to think of supplements like this: God created us and He also created these molecules and compounds that we need to function optimally. And the only way He could figure out to deliver them to us is with these inefficient fruits, vegetables, and animals. But now we, as humans, are so smart that we can bypass this primitive delivery system and get just the little pieces that He intended for us. When I put it like this, it sounds silly, but it is still how a lot of people seem to think.

And this is what the supplement makers want us to think. We no longer think of the benefits of foods, just the constituents. There are hundreds or thousands of compounds in each food and they work together in a very complex manner; but we grossly oversimplify this concept when we think that one isolated compound will have the same effect as the whole food. The argument goes, "Oranges prevent cancer, oranges have vitamin C, so vitamin C prevents cancer and you should take a pill of concentrated vitamin C." This is like, "Cars move people, cars have axles, so I will sell you 1000 axles and you will be able to get around better than someone who only has a car." Foods are put together by nature with the right compounds in the right proportions. If you isolate the compounds, they will not have the same effect as the whole food.

Yin and Yang must balance each other. Whole foods tend to be balanced and in their whole form they have both the Yin and the Yang. Supplements often isolate only one compound and it is usually the Yang aspect. The more you put unbalanced things into your body, the more out of balance it will become.

Now, we can have blood and hair tests, questionnaires, and expert opinions about what you should be taking. The truest test is how it works in you. If you take something and your body functions better, then you probably needed it to-day. That does not mean that you will still need it next week or next year. If you take something for a while and don't notice any difference, you probably didn't need it. Save yourself the money and save your liver having to process it. I like my patients to take as few pills and supplements as possible, but to keep everything that is necessary.

One of the masters with whom I have studied, Dr. Richard Tan from Taiwan says, "My patients always come to me and ask, 'Doc, I have this problem. What should I take for it?' I tell them, 'That is the wrong question. The right question is 'What should you give up?'" I have many patients who are taking handfuls of supplements. One by one they added pills because someone said they should, and now they are on so many that it is impossible to discern which are helping and which are hurting. The natural way to get our Qi is from our food and putting concentrates into our bodies is not a good long-term practice.

One exception to this advice is in regard to chlorella, which are blue-green algae. This is one food we did not take with us when we evolved out of the ocean. It is technically a food, but most people take it in a capsule form. It is still a whole food and it does a great job of providing nutrients and cleaning out impurities in the body, such as heavy metals and other toxins.

Another exception is probiotics. Probiotics are supplements of the bacteria that live in the human digestive tract and aid in digestion. Probiotics are gener-ally only necessary when you are taking antibiotics. Antibiotics kill all bacteria, even the beneficial ones that we need in our body. This can disrupt digestion and cause diarrhea and indigestion. Probiotics replace the good bacteria; but you do not need to supplement the troops when they are not under attack. Under normal circumstances, our bodies should be able to regulate our balance of microorgan-isms and we should not need probiotics.

Herbs

Herbs are a form of supplementation widely utilized in Asia. In America, opinions tend to fall into two camps when it comes to herbs. Some people believe that only a pill can help them and that herbs can do nothing. I find this somewhat amus-ing as most drugs are made from natural sources (mostly plants). For example, a pharmaceutical company will learn that there is a bush in South America which is used to cure headaches. Company scientists will go down and study this plant and try to make a drug that it as close to that plant as they can, but they have to make it a little different in order to be able to patent it. Then they sell it to us. And somewhere along the way, people get the idea, "That plant can't do anything for me. Only the pill that is trying to be like the plant can help me." And again, the compound they try to emulate is always a very yang aspect, thus making the pill unbalanced. (More about Yin and Yang in Chapter 18.)

In the other camp, there are those who think that herbs, like supplements, are safe because they are natural. Lead is natural; mercury, toadstools, and hemlock are natural. So not everything that is natural is safe to ingest. In the oldest recovered herbal text, several of the medicinal herbs were described as being poisonous, if improperly prescribed, so they should not be taken without proper knowledge.

As much as something can help in the right circumstance, it can hurt when used incorrectly. The Chinese see all symptoms are a manifestation of an inner imbalance. Take for instance the symptom of constipation, which can be caused by too much heat in the body and heat dries the stool making it difficult to pass. But constipation can also come from too much cold in the body and cold makes things tighten up and stop moving, in the same way a stream freezes in the winter. If you have hot-type constipation and take a cooling herb or formula, you may find relief. But if your friend has cold-type constipation and takes the same herb, it could make her symptoms even worse. Every symptom can come from at least two different imbalances, which would each require different treatments.

When properly prescribed, herbs are very safe and effective, but to learn how to prescribe correctly takes years to learn and a lifetime to master. I would not trust the recommendations of the clerk at the health-food store, nor the advice-of-the-month in the health magazines.

Herbs are more like food than drugs and have been studied for thousands of years. One of the things I love about working in Oriental Medicine is that everything we use has been tested for so long. You will never find Vioxx® or Phen-fen on an Oriental Medicine practitioner's shelves. Ephedra surprised a lot of people when they learned that it could cause harm. Herbal texts have written for a very long time that ephedra could be dangerous if consumed for too long, or if taken in too high a dose, or taken by persons with particular conditions. But when someone found out that taking a large dose of ephedra could help promote weight loss, they then marketed it, many people began taking it, overdosing, and some people died; so the FDA responded by banning ephedra.

There is a dangerous state of affairs in this country regarding herbal medicines. The analogy I have for this is: if I pour gasoline on myself and light myself on fire, will we outlaw gas? Of course not. When properly prescribed, ephedra can be a very helpful herb for early stage cold and flu, bronchitis, and urine retention; but now it can no longer be used by anyone. Slowly we are becoming in danger of losing access to the natural products that can promote and protect our health, if people misuse them. Then we will have no choice but to go to the pharmaceutical companies for our remedies.

So the goal with Chinese herbal medicine is to find the right blend of ingredients so that the recommended tea will complement the individuals' condition, bringing them back into balance. Once in balance, herbs give way to food and the patient must try to live correctly and maintain good health. In many parts of Asia, herbal tea formulas are often used preventatively to prepare for the change of season.

There are some safety concerns when it comes to herbs. The Western medical community likes to argue that herbs are not safe because we do not know enough about them, an argument with which I totally disagree. **There is no medical system that is better researched or longer-studied than Chinese Medicinal Herbs.** The things we don't know about are the new drugs.

The other area of concern is regarding the quality and purity of the herbs, and it is unfortunately true that the quality control of products from Asia is not always up to American standards. When some products are analyzed, we may find higher-than-allowable levels of lead, mercury, and other undesirable chemicals. Therefore, it is important to know the source of the herbs you are taking and to know that the company from which they are purchased can assure their quality and safety.

Drugs

Western drugs are not necessarily bad. They have their own properties; and the unique blend of actions in a pill could be exactly the right thing to correct a patient's imbalance. For any given drug, we have learned that it may be a good fit for about 20-30% of people taking it; a fair fit for about 50% of people; and a terrible fit for about 20-30% of people. The problem with drugs is that they cannot be customized for those for whom it is not a good fit. In Chinese herbalism, there is a saying: If an herbal formula causes unwanted side-effects, it is clearly not the right formula. However, in the West we accept the fact that drugs have side effects. Wouldn't it be better if we could tweak things so that we only had the desired outcome and no unwanted effects?

In the Chinese understanding, all symptoms are just the body's way of telling us that something is out of balance. Right now we often use pharmaceuticals to ignore and hide the messages that our bodies are giving us. It is obviously time to stop masking the symptoms and rectify the underlying cause.

An alarming trend in pharmaceutical research is the quest for the life-long treatment. HIV is a wonderful example of this. At this time HIV cannot be cured (I don't know that the pharmaceutical companies are even trying anymore), but they have found an expensive cocktail that you can take forever and which will keep you alive. If you sell a cure, you get paid once; with a lifelong treatment, you get paid for the life of the patient. There are many drugs that are being prescribed with no goal of eliminating them. Drugs to control cholesterol, reflux, hypertension, and even hormone therapies are being used this way and I believe this is bad. We should address the cause of the problem, not just mask it with a pill for life.

(For the record, there are many good scientists and doctors doing important work to cure diseases, who are sponsored by the government and private parties. Unfortunately, that is just not the agenda of the very-well-funded drug companies.)

Chapter Eleven

What about Breakfast?

This is the number one question I'm asked when I give this information in talks to patients and groups. By now you know that I generally recommend vegetables, whole grains, and a little of everything else, a little meat, but no dairy. So, what can you eat for breakfast? Vegetables, whole grains, and a little of everything else.

Humans are the only animals that eat certain foods at certain times of the day. I cannot imagine a lion thinking, "I only have Gazelle after 3pm." Again, this peculiarity is not for all humans. In Asia, breakfast looks a lot like lunch and dinner: they eat rice, vegetables, and fish, etc. The only differences are that they will often have rice porridge instead of steamed rice and they may eat more fruit.

I don't know how we developed this list of foods that are considered breakfast foods. Most of them are very unhealthy and none of them include any vegetables. Waffles and pancakes with syrup are basically desserts and cold cereals are processed and served with cold milk (bad). Eggs are OK sometimes, but not with cheese and meat, and not too often. Oatmeal is good, rice porridge is good, cream of wheat is OK, vegetables are good, and fruits are good. A spinach crepe and a veggie omelet are the only common breakfast foods I can think of that really contain any vegetables. Yet **that which is good for us is good at all times of the day.**

If you like to eat cold cereal, don't have it every day, don't always eat the same one, and don't use the same milk. Rice milk, soy milk, almond milk, goat's milk, and walnut milk are all acceptable substitutes for cow's milk, but don't just pick one; use them all in rotation. Breakfast bars are processed, concentrated, and unnatural – so please avoid them. Keep it natural and try to make breakfast more like the other meals.

Chapter Twelve

Feeding our Children

The choices we make for our children are of paramount importance. First of all, they learn their habits from their parents and if we have bad habits, they will learn and carry them into adulthood. But it is also critical because it is in childhood that the foundations of good health are laid down. We can make the following analogy: if a tree grows well in its early days, it will be strong and able to withstand high winds and bitter winters later in its life. If, however, the tree is compromised in its early growth, it will never reach full strength and stability.

When I was younger, I worked as a playground and cafeteria supervisor at my old elementary school and kids either brought their lunch or ate what the school provided. The hot lunches were often processed, fried, or included cheese (most kids have far too much macaroni and cheese). Milk is the only option for a beverage. The lunches of the kids who brought them from home often included: string cheese, raw vegetables with a cream-based dip, peanut butter, jelly, white bread, crackers, cookies, and fruit juice. And, as we have now learned, these choices are all bad! No wonder our kids are getting more obese and less fit.

You should feed your children the way you should feed yourself. Send them with a bowl of rice and some steamed vegetables, a piece of fruit is better than juice, and water is better than milk. A sandwich on whole grain, rye, wheat, or spelt bread is much better than one made of white bread; and put some vegetables on it. There is nothing wrong with a little lunchmeat sometimes. Peanut butter and jelly is not a good staple food. How often do you eat PB&J? Then why should your kids eat it every day?

For infants, breast milk is best for the first year at least, if at all possible; if breast-feeding is not possible, consult the chapter on Dairy for substitutions. Rice porridge (congee) is a good first food to introduce and you should make your own fresh purees of organic vegetables and fruits. Do not serve too much food cold; and avoid things that are too sweet and sticky, like fruit juice.

Chapter Thirteen

Food Preparation and Cooking Methods

Microwaving food is bad

This is going to take a little explaining, so please hang in here with me. A Japanese scientist, Masaru Emoto, wrote a book called *The Hidden Messages in Water*. He took pictures of water droplets just at the point of freezing and sometimes the water would form a beautiful crystal and sometimes it would just turn to plain ice. He found, interestingly enough, that if you wrote the word "beautiful" on a beaker of water, that water would crystallize; but if you wrote "Ugly" it would not. He reproduced these results writing in many different languages. He continued to experiment and found that different expressions created different types of crystals. "Thank you" in English has the same characteristic shape as "Thank you" in Chinese, Japanese, French, German, Italian, etc., but produced a different shape (in all the languages) than the words "Love" or "Happy.". So these ideas, or their energy, affect water and the source of the water also matters. Water from a mountain stream in Switzerland will crystallize; New York City tap water will not; nor will water from a polluted lake. However, after the water has been prayed over by Buddhist monks, it will then crystallize. Our bodies are made up of about 70% water, so the energy of water affects us too. Water that has been microwaved will not crystallize, as its energy has been damaged.

Microwaves are too intense and they destroy the life in the food. You can test this statement yourself: cut a food in half. Microwave one half for one minute and boil the other half in water for one minute. Save them both and see which one goes bad first.

Dr. Emoto also had school children file past two bowls of rice, telling one bowl, "You're good" and the other, "You're bad". The "bad" rice spoiled much faster than the "good" rice. This sounds crazy I know, but it has all been well documented.

Steaming vegetables is better than boiling

A great many of the nutrients are lost when vegetables are boiled, plus it takes longer and uses more power to bring the extra water required to a boil. Steaming vegetables lightly is efficient, healthy, and fast.

It is also fine to sauté your freshly cut vegetables, but don't use too much of any oil to begin with. What kind of oil should you use? They should be natural and fresh and not sprayed from a can. Some people say olive oil is best, some say palm oil. I believe that rotating a variety of different oils is better than sticking with any single one. You can use olive, canola, corn, soybean, coconut, palm, sunflower, safflower, peanut, flax seed, hemp seed oils, all in moderation.

And, of course, do not eat much deep-fried food.

Preparation

The Chinese have developed very efficient ways for preparing food. For instance, it can take 30 minutes or more to bake a chicken breast, but if you cut it into small pieces first, you can stir-fry it in five. Cutting the food first will shorten cooking time and greatly reduce the amount of fuel you need to use (natural gas, propane, electric, wood, etc.), plus, you only need to wash one knife at the end of the meal!

When food is cut into small pieces, it is easy to eat too fast. However, eating with chopsticks forces you to slow down and also allows any excess sauce to drip off. The Chinese used to use forks (in fact, they invented them), but they found that chopsticks are more conducive to eating properly. Many Americans eat Chinese food with a fork and use a spoon to get all the sauce. However, it should be remembered that the sauce is a condiment, not a food, and any extra sauce should be left on the plate. Do not use rice to soak up the sauce either. Keep the rice pristine, on the side.

Cookware is important

Aluminum pans may seem good because they are cheap and lightweight, but they are the worst for cooking as the aluminum leeches out into your food and then into your body. Aluminum toxicity can interfere with the metabolism of calcium, and can cause extreme nervousness, anemia, headaches, gastrointestinal problems, decreased liver and kidney function, memory loss, speech problems, softening of the bones, loss of coordination, and aching muscles. **Get rid of any aluminum cookware you have and don't cook in aluminum foil.** You also shouldn't drink from aluminum cans too much either: Get your beer from a bottle and get sodas out of your life. **Glass, cast-iron, ceramic, and surgical-grade stainless steel are the best cooking surfaces,** and enamel-coated pans are also good.

Storing food

Glass or ceramic containers are the best in which to store food and paper containers work well too. Tupperware is fine for cold foods, since the plastics do not react at cold temperatures; but do not put hot food into plastic containers as the heat can release dioxins into the food, so let it cool down before putting it in a storage container. Absolutely do not microwave food that is wrapped or contained in plastic. This goes for a frozen dinner too; transfer the meal to a ceramic or glass plate before cooking. Frozen dinners are bad for a variety of reasons, but you can at least eliminate the plastic leeching into your food. Some time ago, it was rumored that by freezing Tupperware containers they released dioxins, but that myth has now been debunked.

Refrigeration

As for refrigeration, I have to give it to our Korean brethren. They have made a product called the Kim chi refrigerator that works so very well at keeping things fresh as the temperature is strictly regulated. These refrigerators are expensive (about twice the price of a normal fridge), but they keep vegetables fresh for several days longer than a conventional refrigerator. For instance, an opened bag of organic salad will still be good for one day in our regular fridge; however, in the Kim chi refrigerator a bag of salad will stay fresh and crisp for over a week. It also keeps meat longer. You don't need one, but if you can afford it, I recommend that you buy the biggest Kim chi refrigerator you can find. But always remember not to eat too much cold food.

Chapter Fourteen

Tips for Losing Weight

Adopting the proper balance of foods will help you lose weight if you need to; but here are some additional tips for those who want to speed the process:

Eat breakfast like a king,
lunch like a merchant, and dinner like a pauper.

Breakfast is the most important meal of the day, and it is the one that we often have the most time to digest. It is not good to go to bed with a full stomach and actually it is best if you don't eat for several hours before lying down for sleep.

Walk 1000 steps after each meal.

In my neighborhood, 1000 steps is the circumference of two blocks and takes me about 10 minutes. This practice stimulates digestion and makes sure the food does not just sit in your stomach and rot. If you get into the habit of moving after eating, you will get out of the habit of stuffing yourself to the point where you cannot move.

Rub your stomach along the direction
of the colon for five minutes after eating.

The colon goes up on the right side, over on the top, down on the left side. Rub your belly in circles in this direction for five minutes after eating. This stimulates the second half of digestion, making room for the first half. You don't need to press too far in, but you do want the stimulation to go deeper than the fat and the abdominal muscles.

Fill your stomach half full with food, a quarter full with fluids
(including soup) and leave the last quarter empty for processing.

If you have ever over-stuffed a washing machine, you know that none of the clothes are washed clean. We need room for the food to churn and process and if we over-stuff ourselves, our digestion gets jammed up and we feel slow and heavy.

Chew your food well.

For one thing, this makes food easier to digest and remember the goal is always efficient digestion. This also helps prevent acid reflux and indigestion and it also forces us to slow down. As it takes about 15 minutes for the brain to get the message that the stomach is full, if we eat more slowly, chewing the food well, we will be less likely to overeat.

Do not go hungry.

Starving yourself is one of the best ways to put on fat, for when we do not eat enough the body thinks it is in a crisis situation and works to protect itself. So it stores all available food as fat, lowers our energy level, and increases our appetite. This makes sense and it will help keep you alive if you truly are starving, but it does not help us if we are trying to lose weight. When the body thinks you are starving, it will do all it can to make sure you do not lose or burn anything more than you absolutely have to.

Exercise in the morning.

When your stomach is empty, the body will burn its stored fat, but don't exercise to the point of feeling dizzy or lightheaded. Even if it is not in the morning, you should get some exercise every day.

Eat small red beans (adzuki beans).

These beans have the same caloric value as beef, but they help to eliminate dampness in the body by increasing urination. The Chinese view excess weight as excess dampness, so increasing urination (naturally) can help. However, as with all foods, keep them in moderation.

Eat more bitter foods or herbs.

Bitter foods drain dampness, cool fire, and resolve phlegm and most of us do not get enough of them. Bitter foods can be easily found in the produce section and include kale, mustard greens, dandelion greens, turnip greens, etc., basically any items that are not especially sweet.

Chapter Fifteen

Lifestyle

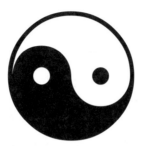

In Chinese culture Yin and Yang represents balance as it is found in nature, though it is not split evenly into black and white. Looking at the symbol above, as we go around the circle, the white part grows until it reaches a maximum, then it fades as black comes in and grows. This is how things change in nature: light in the daytime begins in the morning, reaches a maximum and then gradually fades as night begins. In the same way, summer changes to winter and youth changes to age. There is a dynamic balance of give and take and the more we can emulate nature, the better off we'll be. The same laws govern us, although some people nowadays like to think they are above the laws of nature.

Yin and Yang is a way of understanding all phenomena as lying between two extremes: Yang is the bright, loud, active, masculine, summertime energy of things; and Yin is its complement – soft, quiet, still, feminine, winter, etc. You can't have one without the other.

American culture is all about Yang. We always have to be busy doing something. It is not your fault – you have been brainwashed with this paradigm since you were very young. We keep hearing, "Time is short" "Time is a-wasting," "If you're not moving forward, you're falling behind," "Non-productive time is wasted time," and "I'll rest when I'm dead." We work 50-80 hours a week and then pack our weekends and vacations full of activities. This is an unbalanced lifestyle. If you have a greenhouse, you don't leave the grow lights on 24 hours a day or if you drive an Indianapolis race car, you have to make pit stops to refuel or you won't finish the race.

In America, we are not taught the value of making pit stops; we are told that they are a nuisance and should be avoided or minimized whenever possible. I believe that making pit stops is not taking a break from the game, but rather a necessary piece of the game that should be allowed, appreciated and cultivated.

The Chinese are very good at teaching their children this. Yes, they have to study hard, get straight A's, and excel in their work, but they also have to do their Tai Chi and meditation everyday. This is how life is made sustainable. **We have to cultivate the Yin as well as the Yang.** So try to find more time in your life for things like: meditation, Tai Chi, gentle and restorative yoga, listening to relaxing music, appreciating art, observing nature, etc. These are all good Yin-activities or in-activities. We tend to spend too much of our time "doing" when we should be spending a little more time just "being".

Again, we have the long history of the Asian cultures to thank for this recommendation and, historically, they have tried all sorts of arrangements. For instance, there was an area in China where the people heard about the Spartan lifestyle. These Chinese wondered, "What would happen if we focused on the body? If we ate a lot of protein and worked out all the time?" After some time, they noticed some pretty serious breakdowns, both in the health of the individual and in society. From this experiment they learned, "That doesn't work. Stop that. Tell everyone. And let's figure out how to better re-work this." So, from an historical perspective, they have been through their "type A" phases and found, as we are learning, that that particular lifestyle is a great recipe for burnout. The American 'go-all-the-time' model is great if you want to see how much you can accomplish by the age of 40, but if you want to live well past 40, you need more balance.

Your lifestyle should be balanced and moderate. As noted above, Americans often tend to be an extreme culture and when we do something, we go at it all the way. Over time the Chinese have tried all sorts of arrangements and have found that anything taken to the extreme will eventually pull you out of balance. The Asian ideal is more middle-of-the-road and well rounded. If you stand firmly in the middle of the road, it is hard to be pulled off balance, but if you are dancing on the edge, it doesn't take much to push you over. So the ideal is: don't work too much, don't sleep too much, or play too much, etc.

Exercise

It is also not good to exercise too much. I have some patients who exercise excessively and can't believe that a health care provider would tell them to exercise less. But this is representative of our American mindset, i.e. if a little is good, more must be better.

I had a patient who came in recently and said, "This year I'm going to get in shape." I said, "That's great!." He said, "So I'm going to start running." I said, "Great!" He said, "So I'm going to start running one hour every day." I had to tell him, "That's not great." He had been running zero hours a month and was suddenly going to jump all the way to 30 hours a month. I told him to start slowly, and to include more varied exercises in his exercise program. This patient is typical of our culture – when we do something, we do it to the extreme. We have a lot of muscles that can be worked in many different ways and if we do the same exercises all the time, we overuse some body parts to the exclusion of others. One thing the Chinese do right is that most of them get some exercise every day. Every morning in China, the parks are filled with people practicing their Tai Chi, Qi Gong, Kung Fu, etc. People of all ages, physical abilities, and social classes, spend between 20-60 minutes getting their bodies and minds prepared for the day. Sometimes people will practice a second time either in the middle of the workday or after work; but once a day is still adequate.

The Western medical community recommends 20 minutes of exercise, three times a week and for some people it can be hard to find 20 minutes. For instance, if you go to a gym, that 20 minutes can take more than an hour when you factor in a commute, changing, and showering. But remember, this is not an all-or-nothing proposition and while not everyone may be able find 20 minutes, everyone can find at least one. One minute of exercise is not as much as we need, but it is still better than none. Most people I know shower everyday, so while you are waiting for the water to warm up, knock out a few push-ups, sit-ups and deep knee bends, or lift some dumbbells. Gradually shoot for two minutes a day, and then three, etc. If you do this in the morning, very soon you will find yourself waking with more energy. Also it's important to stretch your joints and muscles regularly and if you watch TV at night (not recommended in excess), sit on the floor and stretch while watching. When you are flexible, you are less prone to injury. Stretching is not just for athletes.

Tai Chi is the best exercise. It is gentle, but can be deceivingly strenuous and it is the only exercise that gives you more energy than you had to begin with. It is a Qi cultivation tool, regarded as essential for people in the field of acupuncture, since we are giving away our Qi all day. Most other exercises are a trade-off; and in general, that is acceptable. "I'll sacrifice this much energy so I can burn this much fat or build this much muscle." But with Tai Chi, you can burn the fat, build the muscle, and still end up with more energy than you had to begin with.

Tai Chi is an internal as well as an external martial art. It is as much about freeing the flow in the heart and the mind as it is about working the body and actually, the physical part is the last piece. The practice of this martial art starts with the mind and heart. So when looking for a class, try to find a teacher who focuses on the internal aspects of Tai Chi as well as the body movements.

One rule connected with the body that most of us are familiar with is: **use it or lose it**. If you stay sedentary, you will lose the ability to move and we have to keep moving and keep active. I remember one time I was riding a bus, and a very overweight woman got on, then got off two blocks later. There may have been other circumstances affecting her inability to walk this short distance, so I shouldn't judge; but I remember thinking, "Maybe that's why she's heavy." If you prove to the body that it needs exercise, it will cooperate with you, but don't overdo it, and go slowly at first. Show your body that you need strength and you will build strength; show it you need endurance and your endurance will grow. This formula also applies to your brain: read something educational once in a while, or take a class, and challenge yourself.

Smoking

Tobacco actually has some medicinal and food uses and people have smoked tobacco for thousands of years. The cigarettes that are sold today are very much removed from the pure tobacco smoked by our ancestors. So many additives and chemicals are added to tobacco today that it is no longer a natural product and much of the adulteration of the tobacco is there specifically to increase its addictiveness. A cigarette or pipe of natural tobacco every now and then will not hurt you; but with the incredible addictiveness of today's cigarettes, most people have a very hard (if not impossible) time smoking only in moderation.

Remember, it is what we do every day that catches up with us. Smoking 20 cigarettes a day is not moderate and will have a cumulative effect. The tar builds up in the lungs, it taxes the heart, it makes us age prematurely, and causes scores of other unnecessary health problems.

For most things, I advocate slow and gentle change but this is not a wise recommendation for quitting smoking. There has to be a drastic shift completely away from smoking and the activities associated with smoking. By trying to slowly taper off the habit, someone will remain addicted and uncomfortable longer.

The physical withdrawal from nicotine lasts about 47-72 hours, and can be extremely unpleasant for some people. Acupuncture can help make this transition much easier, but you have to be ready to quit. If you are not yet ready, please visit the American Lung Association's website (www.lungusa.org) for more motivation. When you are ready, throw away your cigs, ashtrays, lighters, pipes, and all the paraphernalia associated with the habit and start acupuncture on the day that you are going to quit. Avoid the places and activities with which you have associated tobacco and whenever you want a cigarette, brush your teeth. This works better than chewing gum because it satisfies the hand-mouth habit. Even if you have to brush your teeth 20 times a day, that's still better than smoking.

It seems like an oxymoron when smokers say that they find the practice relaxing, for nicotine is a stimulant, so how could it be relaxing? It is the deep inhalation that has this relaxing effect. Breathing deeply makes the blood more alkaline, which in turn has a calming effect on the brain. So when you feel that you need a cigarette, take some deep breaths.

If you fall off the wagon and begin smoking again, you will be re-introducing the physical addiction and will have to go through the withdrawal all over again. Do it! Quit again. Don't give up your previous efforts and resign yourself to remaining a smoker for life.

Sleep

Most of us don't get enough sleep and our culture doesn't even value it. We should sleep for eight hours a night and most of us barely manage six hours. I have heard laudatory reports that Bill Clinton functions on five hours of sleep a night. The report's tone implied that this is a goal to which we all should aspire. I don't believe that this is a good idea. You need to get plenty of sleep in order to work well and the goal is not to be more active more of the time. The goal is to reflect nature and be in step with it; we should be active in the Yang daytime , and restful in the Yin nighttime.

I have patients who sleep 5-6 hours a night, are tired all the time, and ask me how they can stop being so tired. You don't have to be a doctor to figure this one out and if this is your situation, your body is trying to tell you something. Listen to your body, don't ignore it or push it beyond its limits. You need to keep your body well and in shape for a good 100 years, so don't burn it out prematurely.

Between the hours of about 10pm to 6am, the body repairs itself. This is when the maintenance crew comes in; and they can only do their job when the body is at rest and asleep. It is not effective to get your sleep at another time of day and studies have shown that this is why people who work night shifts die at a younger age. When you sleep, try to keep your spine in line as much as possible. You may want to bring a mirror to your bed and try out different pillows to determine which one is the best fit for you. If you sleep on your back, you probably need about one to two inches of pillow support under your head to keep your spine in line. If you sleep on your side, you need four to six inches of support. Sleeping on your side is not as good as sleeping on your back, because on your side, the lower arm is crushed while the upper arm is unsupported. Hugging a pillow can support the upper arm, but the lower arm will still suffer impaired circulation. (Caveat: women who are pregnant should not sleep flat on their backs beyond the first trimester.)

Miscellaneous

Don't carry your wallet in your back pocket as it compresses the sciatic nerve and can cause back and leg pain. I have had many patients (myself included) for whom moving the wallet relieved sciatic pain.

Try to introduce more symmetry into your activities. For example, if you use a computer a lot, try to use your left hand for the mouse some of the time. We are not designed to be in the same position or to be doing the same activity all day.

Make sure you move and change position at least once an hour.

And, lastly, women's shoes are bad for women. I have treated many women whose shoes have injured their feet, ankles, knees, hips, and backs. Please make comfort be at least one of your deciding factors in choosing footwear.

Chapter Sixteen

Attitudes

A lmost everyone in our culture appears to have too much stress in his or her life. Stress taxes the system and causes us to retain weight. So, in addition to being happier, changing attitudes can also help improve the metabolism.

Our attitudes should be balanced and moderate. Life goes up and down and sometimes everything is fine and sometimes things are not so fine; things get harder then and things get easier. This pattern is going to continue for the rest of our lives, possibly following us into the next realm – who knows? So when things are bad, don't get too despondent as nothing lasts forever; nothing ever does and things **will** get better. Similarly, when everything is going great, don't get too comfortable, because life will likely pull the rug out from under you again. And that's OK. It is said that the kid who never falls down, never learns how to get up again; so there is value in being knocked down; and you will always get back up – you always have. There is only one thing in this life that is going to kill you – everything else you will get through, one way or another.

Keep a broad perspective. There have been many times in your life when you have felt overwhelmed with a particular situation, but now you don't even remember it. So next time you feel overwhelmed, take a step back. Instead of worrying, "Oh, my gosh, what am I going to do? Things are never going to be the same again," remind yourself that you have felt that way before and most of those times you have probably completely forgotten. This is because you do make it through everything. So tell yourself, "I don't know how I'm going to get past this, but I'm sure I will, one way or another, because I always have." When you are confronted with a challenge, you can either make it over that mountain or not and either way, you'll be there afterward to learn from it and that is what I think we are here to do.

There is a mindset in our culture that we must accomplish as much as we can in as little time as possible and with the fewest mistakes. I don't buy into that: I believe **we are here to learn and to teach**. We learn from our successes, but we also learn from our mistakes. Sometimes I think that mistakes are the more powerful teachers, so I try to make at least one mistake a day – just so I can learn from it. Sometimes I will even repeat the same mistake over and over again – just to be sure I've really learned from it. In past relationships my pattern was, "Things didn't work out with this girl. Let's find another one just like her and see how things go." I know I'm not alone in making that mistake.

Sometimes it may take us five or ten times of reaching in one direction and having our wrists slapped before we learn that that was not the right way for us to go. It does not mean that the third time was wasted; it simply got us closer to the fifth or tenth time, so it all has value. At some point there may be a quantum shift in our thinking and behavior and until then, we keep getting closer to changing. We are always learning.

And we are always teaching. We like to think that we lead by example and that people can learn from how great we are. But some of the most important teachers in our lives are the bad examples – the ones who modeled behavior and when we saw it we thought, "That's ugly. I don't want to be like that." So we can be grateful for the ignorant, petty, mean, and jerky people in our lives. They help us to see how we **don't** want to be. We learn from our mistakes, and others learn from ours as well.

The Chinese are ahead of us as they take a broader perspective, because Buddhism has long been a part of their culture. Buddhists believe in reincarnation. So as small as one day appears compared to an entire lifetime, when you multiply that by 500 lifetimes, each day of this current lifetime is truly just a drop in the bucket. As a Buddhist I can say, "My girlfriend dumped me. Big deal. I've lost wives, and husbands, and children before. And I will again. This is just another thing from which I can learn." But even if you believe in only one lifetime, as many of us in the West do, this lifetime is still pretty long. What happens today can possibly ruin your day. It might even ruin your week, but your year will probably be OK, and the decade will probably be just fine.

So **life is just a series of challenges designed to help us learn things**. Granted, it's annoying and inconvenient and most of us would like to set up this wave and ride it until we die, but that's not what we are faced with here. And, in the absence of challenges, I might as well die, because I would no longer be learning and developing anyway.

There are some sects of Buddhism that believe a child's spirit can choose its parents. When a child is going to be born handicapped or deformed, the spirits will vie for that body, as there are some lessons that can only be learned through those particular challenges that cannot be learned in a healthy body. So **try to see the challenges in your life as blessings** and as opportunities for growth. Remember, the kid who never falls down, never learns to get up. The person who has to lift 100 pounds will become stronger than the person who only has to lift 10 pounds.

The fact that we are here indicates to me that we have more to learn; we are not yet enlightened, we are not yet one with God; we are not yet in heaven, or whatever paradigm you like. So it is understandable and very forgivable when we mess up. I believe what we're all doing here is trying to figure this all out. So cut yourself some slack and, by extension, we also have to cut some slack for our fellow travelers. **We are all at different stages of our spiritual evolution** – some of us may have further to go than others. So when you encounter people who are ignorant, petty, or jealous, etc., don't look at them with contempt or disdain, rather look at them with compassion. Try to think, "I'm sorry that you are struggling with this, and I hope you find a way over this soon. But I don't want to get pulled into your struggle, because I have my own issues I have to work on. Good luck." Not that we should be cold and indifferent – we should try to have compassion for all creatures (including jerks). But sometimes we need to have boundaries, for if someone's energy is toxic, maybe we need to insulate ourselves from them. If someone is about to make a mistake, maybe they need to make that mistake in order to learn.

Don't listen too much to what others tell you about what you should be doing; all of us are at least partly in the dark. Those people who tell you that you are not living the right way should probably spend more time focusing on themselves. The right path for your enlightenment is going to be different from everyone else's, for as the Buddha says, "Do not walk where I walked, but seek what I sought." I believe that each of us has a piece of the Divine within us. So we need to trust that and listen to our inner wisdom.

Your emotions should be like the wind – felt when they are here, and not when the event has passed. I have worked with some people whose whole day could be ruined if someone cut them off while they were driving to work. It might make some sense to be angry at the time, but hours later when you are in a completely different setting, it doesn't make sense to hold on to that feeling. You are no longer in that situation. There is no shortage of stress – so you don't need to cling to today's stress. There is always more fresh stress coming, so let go of the past, it cannot be changed and don't let it continue to bother you. All we can do is try and learn from it and move on. Be where you are now. I wrote a song about this called *Little Challenges* and you can listen to it at: www.myspace.com/jasonbussell.

Here is a nice story from the Buddhist sutras:

> *A monk and his apprentice were traveling across the countryside. This particular sect of Buddhism was prohibited from having any contact with women. At one point, a woman approached them and*

pleaded, "Please, can you help me across the river? I have medicine that my sister needs or she will die, and I cannot cross the river myself. Please, will you help me?"

At first, the monk ignored her, but she continued to plead for help. The monk dropped his walking stick, picked her up and carried her across the river. He set her down on the other side, crossed back, picked up his walking stick and began walking along their path again. The apprentice was very disturbed by this. He did not say anything, but it stayed in his mind as they continued to walk.

At the end of the day's journey, they set up camp. The apprentice was still visibly upset, so the master asked, "Do you have something on your mind?" The apprentice said, "Yes. Yes I do. That woman today. How could you do that? We're not supposed to have anything to do with women, but you did. Not only did you talk to her, but you touched her and you carried her. How could you do that?" The master chuckled and said, "My dear apprentice, I only carried her for one minute. Have you been carrying her around with you all day?"

We should try to live in the moment as we only get one chance at each moment. If we spend this one completely consumed with what has happened in the past or what may happen in the future, we will miss this moment forever. (For more on this, see Eckhart Tolle's *The Power of Now*.)

Don't overestimate your sphere of influence. We are mostly in control of ourselves – mostly and that's about it. We cannot control our family, friends, significant others, bosses, traffic, weather, etc., and if we think we can, we will drive ourselves, and those around us, crazy. Control can be a comforting delusion, but it is not possible. So we do what we can and we see what happens. And whatever happens, it's OK.

Anxiety usually has a component of needing to control things. "If I am vigilant enough, I can make sure that nothing bad ever happens." Well, I'm sorry to inform you that bad things are going to happen. They are supposed to, for it is going through the hard times that make the good times so good. The key is not to prevent bad things from happening but to reframe our thinking so we no longer perceive that bad things are bad; they are just part of the smorgasbord of events with which life presents us.

Don't be too quick to judge. In America, we tend to be very quick to judge yet we never know ahead of time how a situation is going to turn out. There is never an end-of-game where they tally up the points, so there is no point in trying to keep score of what was good and what was bad. History is rife with examples of situations that seemed to be bad at the time but, in fact, turned out well in the end.

There is a famous Chinese proverb that illustrates this lesson.

"A Chinese farmer has a stallion. One day the stallion runs away.
The village people come to him and say, "Ah, such bad luck!"
The farmer shrugs, "Good luck, bad luck, who knows?"

A few days later the stallion returns with three mares. The village
people come to him and say, "Ah, such good luck!"
The farmer shrugs, "Good luck, bad luck, who knows?"

The next day, the farmer's son is out trying to tame the mares. One
of them kicks him and breaks his leg. All the neighbors sympathize
with the farmer's bad luck, but the farmer is still not convinced.

A week later, government officials come to the town and draft all
the young men to fight in the army. The farmer's son is not drafted
because he has a broken leg.

And so on it goes. . ."

I believe that **fate makes no mistakes**. If something happens, it is de-facto what was supposed to happen. So it doesn't make sense to spend too much time dwelling on the coulds and shoulds, because that is not reality-based – it is fantasy. We all love to fantasize about how things could have gone differently for us, but those are just ... fantasies. For instance, I like to fantasize about winning the lottery. But what I don't know is that if I did win, I might be on the highway, on the way to cash in my ticket, and a truck hits my car and kills me. We never know how things might have turned out differently, so we must accept where we are and go from there.

Women in this country are socialized to be givers and, following role models such as June Cleaver and Carol Brady, they are expected to put their own needs last. If they do anything for themselves, they then feel they are being selfish and thoughtless. I think this is terrible. If you are not well, you are no good to anyone else. The Chinese are always thinking in terms of balance, so I quote them a lot. There also is an ancient Hebrew text which asks, **"If I don't act for myself, who** will? If I act only for myself, what am I? If not now, when?" Both traditions point to the need for balance.

There is a growing awareness of the idea of Karma in our culture. In the Buddhist tradition, Karma is that which balances all. It is often loosely translated as, "What goes around, comes around." The more good you put out in the world, the more good will be reflected back to you; Likewise, the more negativity you give out, the more negativity will be reflected back to you. There is also something else about Karma that most people overlook, which is that **it is good Karma to help other people develop their Karma**. If you are always giving and never taking, you are hoarding all the good Karma, so we should remember that other people like to feel useful and helpful too. If we never let people help us, we deprive them of their spiritual growth. Of course this can be taken too far and we do not want to take advantage of the kindness of others, because no one will like us. However, we don't need to be too concerned with what others think of us: it's all about balance.

Try to find the humor in life. Life is full of irony and coincidences and almost never turns out the way we would expect. The Buddha (which means "enlightened person" and you do not have to be Buddhist to be a Buddha) goes through life with a sense of mild bemusement. We should all enjoy the dance and appreciate the intricacies of life, but not get too wrapped up in it, nor too invested in any one outcome – for that is a sure recipe for disappointment.

To change our attitudes takes practice and at first that may feel unnatural. However, I would like to challenge you to view this as a debate. As you know, debate is the sport of arguing and in a debate match, each team has to "argue" one side of an issue and neither team gets to pick which side to "argue"; each team has to defend their given position, whether or not they believe in it. Lawyers have to do this all the time. So I challenge you to be your own devil's advocate. Many of us have well-rehearsed scripts of worry and guilt that seem to play automatically when triggered. When that happens, try to argue against that script: "Wait a minute, is there another way to look at this?" With time and practice this will become more natural and soon all the glasses you see will be half full, not half empty.

Age does not necessarily bring wisdom with it. However, the longer we live, the more chances we have to learn the lessons, but we all know some people who have lived to a ripe, old age but are still very closed minded and inflexible in their thinking. When I graduated from college, I had some post-baccalaureate hubris and thought I knew it all; plus, I thought that to change my mind would be to admit I had been wrong. Then one day I saw a bumper sticker that changed my life and it read "If you can't change your mind, how are you sure you still have one?" This got me thinking and I realized that the minute we believe we know it all is the minute we stop learning. And then we might as well be dead. So as long as we are here, we need to keep an open mind and keep learning.

The following is a passage from the Tao Te Ching, the foundation text of Taoism. Reading and understanding this book can lead to serenity and peace, so I give this particular passage to a lot of my patients (please forgive the gender-specificity of it).

Man is born gentle and supple.

At his death he is hard and stiff.

Green plants are tender and filled with sap.

At their death they are withered and dry.

Therefore the stiff and unbending is the disciple of death.

The gentle and yielding is the disciple of life.

An army without flexibility never wins a battle.

A tree that is unbending is easily broken.

The hard and strong will fall.

The soft and yielding will overcome.

[Tao Te Ching, 76]

Chapter Seventeen

Summary

So that's it, you have now read all the main points I wished to make on how Asian culture, its philosophies and its diet can improve health. I have given talks on this subject enough times to know that people hear what they want to hear and often overlook important aspects of this advice. Therefore, I recommend that you go through and re-read all this material. I have purposely kept the book short and manageable so that you can read it several times and really understand the concepts. But to make it easier, here are the highlights:

- Balance and moderation are the keys
- Eat mostly whole grains, cooked vegetables, and a little of everything else (except dairy)
- White rice is the best but should not be taken to the exclusion of the other grains
- Simpler foods are easier to digest, avoid processed foods
- Avoid artificial sweeteners
- Cooked vegetables are better than raw
- Cold and refrigerated foods are unnatural and impair our digestion
- Eat a wide variety of vegetables, especially those grown locally and in season
- Vegetables are better than fruit, which should be taken in moderation
- Juice is not moderate and should therefore be limited
- Eat a little of all types of meat: fish (fresh and salt-water, shellfish), fowl (white and dark meat), and mammal (different parts of different animals). Too much or too little is not good
- Avoid dairy! Milk and its derivatives are for infants. Cows' milk is for calves and is NOT healthy, despite what the commercials "teach"
- Chew food thoroughly
- The stomach should be filled half way with food, a quarter way with fluid (including soup), and a quarter left empty for processing
- Drink at least one cup of green tea every day

- Exercise body and mind a little every day. Don't overdo it and don't always do the same exercise
- Don't worry about things; everything turns out OK in the end. Just try to learn from life.
- Don't overestimate your personal sphere of influence
- Be patient and compassionate
- Don't be too quick to judge
- Find the humor in life
- Change slowly for the better

If we follow these guidelines, we will all be much healthier and happier. There is no need to worry about calories, carbs, fat, or any of those trends; just adhere to the principles of the Asian Diet and all will be well.

What follows is an introduction to Oriental Medicine and the understood actions of common food. I invite you to educate yourself about these fields also. And going back to re-read the first part of the book again is a really good idea

Chapter Eighteen

Basics of Oriental Medicine

I n order to understand Asian Dietary Therapy, you should learn a little about Asian Medical Theory. Asian medicine, like Asian philosophy is all about balance. Finding and maintaining balance is the goal of life. If you are in balance, you should have no undesirable symptoms. If you have symptoms, that means that you are out of balance. A simple example of this is: if you have a fever, you have too much heat in the body; if you have chills, you have too much cold. It gets a lot more complicated than this, but it is important to remember that all pathologies can be interpreted as some type of imbalance.

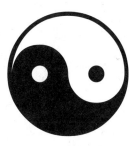

Yin and Yang

The above symbol is the Tai Chi symbol; also known as the Yin-Yang symbol. This represents balance as it is found in nature.

Yin-Yang theory is a way of understanding all phenomena as lying between two extremes. Yin and Yang are interdependent and neither can exist without the other. They define each other, they complement each other, they balance each other, and they transform into each other. If you travel North long enough, you'll end up heading South; likewise, if you stay up late enough in the evening, it will become early morning. Everything in nature can be described as Yin or Yang in comparison to its opposite. The following chart illustrates this.

Yin	Yang
Down	Up
Cold	Hot
Front	Back
Female	Male
Substantial	Energetic
Winter	Summer
Internal	External
Quiet	Loud
Soft	Hard
Night	Day
Inactive	Active
Moist	Dry

As I have said before, in its simplest form Asian medicine is about balancing Yin and Yang.

The Five Phases

Yin and Yang is a simple way of categorizing the world, but the Chinese recognized more intricate relationships and developed the theory of five phases (also known as five elements) to further describe and understand the world. The five phases are: wood, fire, earth, metal, and water; and their relationships are understood as being both promoting and controlling.

In the Sheng, or generating, cycle (the curved arrows), Wood gives rise to Fire (Wood burns), Fire gives rise to Earth (ashes), Earth gives rise to Metal (Metal is

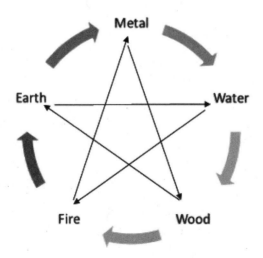

found in the earth), Metal gives rise to Water (the way dew condenses on a metal plow), Water gives rise to Wood (it feeds plants). If any of these components is deficient or excessive, it affects the whole cycle. These relationship cycles are understood as mother-child.

In the Ke, or controlling, cycle (the straight arrows), Wood controls Earth (it can overgrow land), Fire controls Metal (it can melt it), Earth controls Water (providing boundaries and passageways), Metal controls Wood (as an axe), and Water controls Fire (which I think is pretty obvious). Again, if one element is too weak or strong, it affects the element that needs to be controlled, and too much or too little control can be problematic. This is considered the grandmother-grandchild relationship. To further complicate matters, the grandchild can act out against the grandmother in what is called the Wu, or rebellion, cycle.

Everything can be classified into a five phase theory as well.

The five phase theory can become extremely complicated and it's not necessary to learn it. The only thing to remember is that flavors have different actions and they, like all things, must be balanced. The foods that we put into our bodies will pull us in different directions. Whether or not we are aware of it, we are affecting our balance with every meal, so we should be very conscious of our food choices.

To clarify the five flavors: the first three are Sweet, Salty, and Sour. Then there is Acrid, which includes the spicy and the aromatics (like garlic and onion). Lastly, there is Bitter, which includes basil, lettuce, parsley, vinegar, tea, and coffee. Most foods are a combination of two or more tastes.

The Sweet flavor harmonizes and moistens, but too much Sweet causes dampness and obesity. Acrid flavor strengthens the Lung, opens the pores to dispel pathogens, and moves things outward and upward (including mood). Too much Acrid can cause overheating and dryness, restlessness, and constipation. Salty flavor supplements the kidneys, leads downward, and dissolves hard lumps in the body. Too much Salty flavor dehydrates, damages fluids, harms the cardiovascular system and causes stiffness in the body and mind. Sour flavor goes to the Liver, and is an astringent. Think about sucking a lemon – what happens to your mouth? It tightens up, which is what is meant by astringent. Sour flavor controls excessive perspiration and urination and because it holds things in, it should not be taken when fighting a cold or virus. Bitter flavor directs things downward, clears heat, and calms; but too much bitter can cause diarrhea and disturb the spirit.

The Organs

The Chinese recognize a different functionality in our internal organs, so please do not confuse the organs I describe with their functions, as understood in the

	Wood	Fire	Earth	Metal	Water
Direction	East	South	Center	West	North
Yin Organ	Liver	Heart	Spleen	Lung	Kidney
Yang Organ	Gall Bladder	Small Intestine	Stomach	Large Intestine	Urinary Bladder
Season	Spring	Summer	Late Summer	Autumn	Winter
Weather	Wind	Heat	Damp	Dry	Cold
Flavor	Sour	Bitter	Sweet	Acrid	Salty
Sense Organ	Eyes	Tongue	Mouth	Nose	Ears
Tissues	Sinews	Vessels	Flesh	Body hair	Bone
Emotion	Anger	Joy	Pensiveness	Sorrow	Fear
Development	Birth	Growth	Maturity	Withdrawal	Ending
Action	Growth, bending	Warming, flaring upward	Ripening, fertility	Reflection, death	Flowing, cooling

West. If your acupuncturist tells you that you have a kidney deficiency, he/she is probably not talking about the function of your Western kidney. We are talking here about the kidney function as understood in the East. In the earliest writings, organs were divided into two kinds: Yang organs (hollow receptacles like the stomach, urinary bladder, gall bladder, and the small and large intestines) and Yin organs (solid and doing work; like the liver, spleen, kidney, heart, and lung). Contrary to popular conception, the lung is not an empty bag but is more like a sponge. The more important organs are the Yin organs.

The liver is in charge of "free-coursing"- i.e., keeping things flowing smoothly. It is considered Wood in the five phases and corresponds to the sour flavor. It governs the sinews (connective tissue) and opens to the eyes. It also stores the blood.

The lungs bring the air into the body and disperse air and fluids. Lungs are Metal in the five phases and corresponds with acrid flavor. It governs the waterways of the body, the skin, and body hair and opens to the nose. As the highest organ in the body, it is the umbrella, protecting the other organs. This is why illness tends to affect the lungs first (lungs include throat and nose).

The kidneys store our reproductive and youthful essence; and are the root of all Yin and all Yang. As the lowest organ in the body, it is the foundation; it also brings the air from the Lungs into the rest of the body. The kidneys represent the Water phase and correspond to the salty flavor. They govern the bones and the two orifices of elimination (front and rear), engender marrow, and open to the ears.

The heart governs the movement of blood and it is the mansion of the spirit. It is the Fire phase and corresponds to the bitter flavor. It governs the vessels and opens to the tongue.

The spleen is the main organ of digestion. The stomach is analogous to the pot, while the spleen is considered the burner. The stomach holds the material while the spleen works on it and is in charge of transporting and transforming the food into useful tissue and energy, or into waste. The taste that corresponds to the spleen is sweet; and its element is Earth and its essence is Qi. The spleen also governs the blood, muscles, and opens to the mouth.

Why do we crave sweets? The taste that corresponds with the Spleen is Sweet. A little sweet flavor can boost the spleen and help its function and this is why we often crave dessert after a meal as it helps jump-start the digestion. But too much sweet is difficult to digest. When we put sugar in a pot and heat it, it gets very sticky. So the spleen has the task of transforming this sticky mess into energy or tissue. This is very difficult, and so the spleen seems to ask for more help (sweet), but this can become a vicious cycle. If you keep over-burdening your stomach and spleen, then your body will keep asking for more and more sweets. However, if you give yourself time to process all the difficult-to-digest

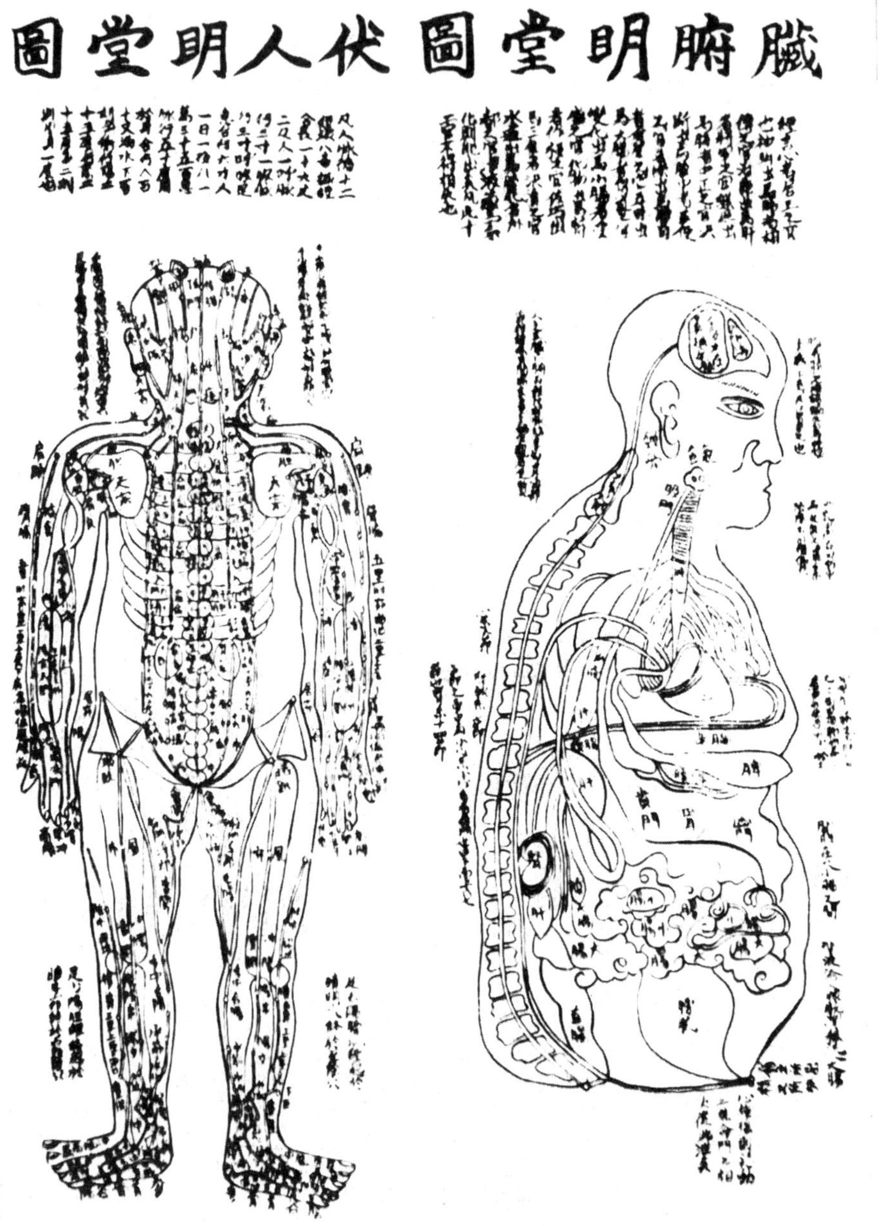
臟腑明堂圖
伏人明堂圖

sweets in your system, your body will stop asking for a boost and this change can happen in less than a week.

As for the Yang organs, the gall bladder is paired with the Liver and represents the Wood phase. It is in charge of decision making.

The stomach is Earth and is paired with the spleen. It is in charge of ripening and rotting the food to prepare it for transformation into Qi.

The small intestine is paired with the heart in the Fire phase. It separates the clear from the turbid in terms of food and liquid.

The urinary bladder is paired with the kidney in the Water phase. It holds the urine. Its channel traverses the back and its acupoints are often used in treating back pain.

The large intestine is the Metal phase and is paired with the lung. It holds the feces, which are transformed by the spleen and expelled by the kidney.

So the main point here is that each flavor feeds a particular organ, and each organ has distinct functions. For this reason, there must be a balance between the five flavors. It can't be all sweet, as that will pull us out of balance.

Qi and blood

One of the most important concepts in Asian medicine is the concept of Qi (pronounced Chee in Chinese). Qi loosely translates as our "Vital Energy." It flows within us and around us. It gives all things life, animation, warmth, and containment, and is like 'the Force' in *Star Wars*. Qi is also known as Prana in the yogic tradition.

We know how the blood flows because we can see it. Autopsy can show exactly where the vessels lead and how much blood they contain. Qi is not substantial and it cannot be seen, so the mapping of its flow was a much greater challenge, yet the Chinese have managed to map the way the Qi flows around the body. Western science has trouble with the concept of Qi and even though we cannot see it, we can see its effects. My wife was once in a discussion with a skeptical doctor at a dinner party. He said to her, "You show me a test-tube full of Qi and I'll believe in it." She said, "OK, then can you show me a test-tube full of love or fear? Are you going to tell me that these things don't affect our physiology?" He stopped arguing and that response is the best I have ever heard given to someone who doubted the importance of Qi.

We get most of our Qi (70%) from the food that we eat, so it is very important that we feed ourselves well. Our stomach holds the food while the spleen acts on it. The Chinese refer to this function as "rotting and ripening" the food and transforms it into Qi. Then, in turn, we disperse and diffuse the Qi and energy.

The good, usable nutrition goes to the tissues and the turbid waste goes to the toilet. We basically act as filters for the food and we want to make this function as minimally taxing as possible.

The Chinese concept of **Blood** is similar to how we understand it in the West. It nourishes the tissues, but it also calms and cools. Improper diet can lead to a blood-deficiency and people with deficient blood tend to be pale, thin, and sickly, have irregular menstruation and difficulty conceiving, irritable, and have trouble sleeping. Qi and blood are a Yin-Yang pair. Can you guess which is Yin and which is Yang?

Meridians

The channels along which the Qi flows are called Meridians and there are 12 main channels with each one flowing into the next and into the next in a continuous closed circuit. There are also smaller network and capillary vessels to carry the Qi to every cell in the body. Where there is no Qi, there is no life. When the Qi is flowing in harmony, the body is in a natural state of good health – there is no pain, digestion is efficient, and mood is appropriate, etc. This is how we were designed to function. For a variety of reasons, however, this flow of Qi can become disrupted, which causes a myriad of symptoms.

Acupuncture

Acupuncture is the insertion of very thin, sterile needles into influential points on the meridians (acupoints) in order to affect and balance the flow of Qi in the body. The meridian system can be thought of as a system of rivers through which the Qi flows. For a variety of reasons, that flow can be come disrupted, which can be caused by diet, lifestyle, attitudes, environment, heredity, or a host of other factors. When this happens, it is like a tree falling and damming a river; where there was once clear, flowing water, the river can start to back up and become murky and turbid. The riverbanks swell and there is an excess of water upstream of the dam, while downstream there is a lack of water. Acupuncture can be thought of as the process of lifting these trees and unblocking the channel, so that the body can return to a state of balance. The meridian system can also be thought of as a circuit board in the body: throwing a switch in one part of the body affects the energy flow in another.

Each channel connects with, and is named for, an internal organ. In my town, there is a street called Lake Street, which goes to Lake Michigan. Now, there is a lot more to Lake Street than the place where it touches the lake. But if you want to go to the lake, Lake Street is a good way to get there. This is similar to the names of the meridians: there is a lot more to the lung channel than just the lung, including its overall function and the area that it traverses.

Qi is the most primal communication system in the body. When we are just four cells in our mother's womb, those cells communicate via Qi. As we develop, the other systems (circulatory, respiratory, muscular, nervous, digestive, etc.) are built upon that foundation. We can think of it like a house: if the foundation is not aligned, then all that is built upon it can be compromised. However, if we bring the foundation into alignment, all that is built upon it should fall back into its proper place.

But acupuncture is not the only way we can affect the Qi. Everything we do affects it. The three greatest factors that get us out of balance are our diet, lifestyle and attitudes. The typical American is usually out of balance in all three areas, and most people don't even seem to care and treat their bodies like a tool, or an object to be used and abused. Our bodies give us messages all the time but many of us don't listen. We are uncomfortable after we eat too much, but we continue to overeat. It hurts when we play too much tennis, so we try to figure out a way we can still play too much tennis but hurt ourselves less. We have a severe disconnect between the way we treat our bodies and how our bodies behave. If you put cheap gas in your car and it started breaking down, you would then use better gas. Your body is breaking down and yet you continue to give it the same gas. (I assume your body is functioning sub-optimally in at least some way or you would not be reading this book). We need to re-establish the connection between how we treat our bodies and how they act.

The six external pathogens

The Chinese understand that the way things work outside the body is how they work inside the body. So the things that happen in nature happen in us. The six pathogens, or imbalances, that can get into us are: Heat, Cold, Dryness, Dampness, Wind, and Summer-heat (Summer-heat is very rarely seen in the West).

Heat can manifest many ways: it can dry the stool and cause constipation, but it can also agitate the intestines and cause diarrhea. It can cause a red face, hypertension, red eyes, swollen and painful joints. It can cause the blood to boil and leak out, for instance with nosebleeds, excessive menstruation, or breakthrough bleeding. Heat can also lead to anxiety, insomnia, fever, hot phlegm, red rashes, and much more.

Cold can cause rigidity, chills, constipation or diarrhea, runny nose, cough, poor circulation, white rashes, loss of appetite, cancer, phlegm, frequent urination, and more.

Dryness can cause constipation, dry rashes, dry eyes, dry mouth, difficulty urinating, insomnia, brittle nails, and dry cough, amongst other problems.

Dampness can cause diarrhea, edema, weepy rashes, excessive salivation and tears, phlegm, cough, runny nose, sinus problems, etc. The Chinese understand excess weight as excess dampness in the body.

Phlegm is what happens to dampness when it stops moving and congeals. Phlegm can cause obesity, respiratory problems, sinusitis, rhinitis; it can also cause a mental fog and contribute to forgetfulness and Alzheimer's disease. It can congeal to form cancer, and other growths can also be caused by congealed phlegm.

Wind comes and goes mysteriously, and it makes things shake. Wind in the body can cause pain, spasms, Parkinson's disease, stroke, facial paralysis, and much more. Also, other pathogen can ride into the body on the wind, so you can have wind-cold, wind-heat, wind-damp, wind-dryness, and wind-phlegm.

In addition to the external pathogens, we can engender our own internal pathogens through improper diet and thinking. Too much sweetness can cause dampness, too much worry can cause stagnation, etc. So, all things must be in balance.

Stagnation is a lack of flow and can be physical or mental. Tumors, swellings, and pain can all be manifestations of stasis. Depression, anxiety, and anger are also types of stagnation, such as getting stuck on a particular thought. Much therapy in Chinese medicine is aimed at resolving stagnation.

Most symptoms can arise from at least two different imbalances or pathogenic factors. The common cold can either be in a cold-phase (chills, runny nose with thin-clear discharge), or in a hot-phase (fever, sweating, thick-yellow phlegm). So it is not enough to know the symptoms, you also have to discern the cause. With herbal medicine, an improper diagnosis could lead to a treatment that makes the condition worse (treating the common cold, hot-phase, with warming herbs). Food therapies are safer and gentler, but it is important to start paying more attention to the ways that symptoms manifest and try to understand them in terms of these pathogenic factors.

Treatment principles

Treatment in Chinese medicine can seem simple, but it is also commonsense. For instance, in a dry condition, the treatment principle is to moisten. Heat should be cooled and dampness either drained or transformed. If there is vomiting, then we want to direct the Qi downward, but if there is diarrhea or frequent urination, then we want to direct the Qi upwards. The rule is clear: that which is in excess should be reduced and that which is deficient should be supplemented. In the next chapter, the actions of foods are described in terms such as these.

Chapter Nineteen

Actions of Common Foods

In the following list, for each food, I have noted: a) the taste and temperature classification; b) the channels that the food's energy enters; and c) its known functions and applications. The average Asian person knows many of these attributes and actions, as they have been learned from their mothers. You will notice that the attributes directly correlate to the action: cool foods treat heat conditions; moistening foods treat dry conditions, and so on. Since we know the *effect* of different tastes, knowing these tastes gives us clues as to the food's actions. And since we know the *functions* of the different organs, understanding the channels through which the food enters also points to the actions of the food. It is not necessary to remember these, but this list can be used as a resource. I challenge you to try and get as many of these foods into your diet at least once in the next year.

Abalone
Sweet, Salty, Neutral temperature. Enters the liver and kidney channels.
Enriches Yin, clears heat, replenishes essence, and brightens the eyes.
Treats vaginal discharge and bleeding, dry cough, urinary problems, and cataracts.

Alcohol
Bitter, Sweet, Acrid and Warm. Enters the heart, liver, stomach and lung channels.
Clears heat in the lungs.
Treats cough and hemorrhoids.

Alfalfa Sprout
Bitter and Cool. Enters the spleen, stomach and large intestine channels.
Dries dampness, clears heat from the Stomach, eases urination and defecation.
Treats edema and kidney stones.

Almond
Sweet and Neutral. Enters the lung and large intestine channels.

Moistens the Lung, moves the stool.
Treats panting and dry-type constipation.

Anise

Acrid, Sweet and Warm. Enters spleen, kidney and liver channels.
Warms Yang, moves the Qi, frees the stool and urine.
Treats low back pain, constipation and abdominal distention.

Apple

Sweet and Cool. Enters the lung, stomach and large intestine channels.
Engenders fluids, moistens the lung, and calms the spirit.
Treats hangover, indigestion, morning sickness, and chronic enteritis.

Apricot

Sweet, Sour and Neutral. Enters the spleen, stomach, lungs, and large intestine
    channels.
Moistens the lung, engenders fluids, and relieves thirst.
Treats dry throat and dry-type constipation.

Asparagus

Sweet, Bitter and Cold. Enters the lung, spleen and kidney channels.
Clears heat, drains dampness, and clears the lungs.
Treats excessive thirst, skin eruptions, scanty lactation, and constipation.

Bamboo Shoots

Sweet, Slightly Bitter, and Cold. Enters the lung, large intestine and stomach
    channels.
Clears heat, transforms phlegm, harmonizes digestion, and moistens intestines.
Treats measles and discharge of mucus.

Banana

Sweet and Cool. Enters the lung and large intestine channels.
Clears heat, moistens intestines, and counteracts toxins.
Treats hemorrhoids, constipation, alcoholism, and excessive thirst.

Barley

Sweet, Salty, and slightly cool. Enters the spleen, stomach, and gall bladder channels.
Clears heat, eliminates dampness, cools the blood, boosts the Qi, nourishes blood,
    and frees urination.

Treats diarrhea, edema, pain in urinating, burns, indigestion, and jaundice.

Basil
Acrid and Warm. Enters the lung, spleen, stomach, and large intestine channels.
Dispels cold and dampness, moves the Qi.
Relieves abdominal distention and some types of headaches, menstrual problems, Stomach gas and diarrhea.

Beef
Sweet and Neutral. Enters the spleen, liver, kidneys, stomach and large intestine channels.
Replenishes Qi and blood, Yin and fluids. Strengthens bones and joints.
Treats emaciation, excessive thirst, diabetes, low back and/or knee pain.

Beet
Sweet and Neutral. Enters the heart and liver channels.
Nourishes and moves the blood, moistens intestines, and regulates the menses.
Treats chest congestion and poor energy circulation.

Bell Pepper (green or red)
Acrid and Hot. Enters the heart and spleen channels.
Warms the interior, promotes digestion, and increases appetite.
Treats vomiting, diarrhea, and abdominal pain.

Black Pepper
Acrid and Hot. Enters the stomach and large intestine channels.
Warms the center, resolves phlegm, and food stagnation.
Treats vomiting, cold abdominal pain, cold-type diarrhea, and indigestion.

Broccoli
Sweet, slightly Bitter, and Cool. Enters the spleen, stomach and bladder channels.
Clears heat, frees urination, brightens the eyes.
Treats redness of the eyes and difficult urination.

Buckwheat
Sweet and Cool. Enters the spleen, stomach and large intestine channels.
Opens the stomach, loosens intestines, relieves food stagnation, and diarrhea.
Treats food stagnation, diarrhea, flat abscesses on the upper back and scalding burns.

Burdock root (Yes, you can cook with this root. Peel, julienne, and add to stir-fry.)
Acrid, Bitter, and slightly Cold. Channels entered not yet known.
Clears heat, resolves toxins, fights cancer, and toxic sores.
Treats toxic heat and red, ulcerated sores.

Cabbage
Sweet, slightly Bitter, and Cool or Neutral. Enters the spleen, stomach and small intestine channels.
Clears blood and strengthens the stomach.
Treats constipation in women and the elderly. Relieves spasms and pain.

Cantaloupe
Sweet, Aromatic, and Cool. Enters the lung, heart, large intestine, small intestine, and bladder channels.
Clears heat, moistens dry Lungs, and disinhibits urination.
Treats fever with thirst, dry cough and dry-type constipation.

Cardamom
Acrid, Aromatic, and Warm. Enters the stomach and spleen channels.
Transforms dampness, quiets restless fetus, and harmonizes the stomach.
Treats nausea, indigestion, vomiting, morning sickness, and helps stabilize a threatened miscarriage.

Carp
Sweet and Neutral. Enters the spleen and kidney channels.
Directs downward, opens the water passages, improves lactation, and reduces swelling.
Treats edema, beriberi, jaundice, cough, and insufficient lactation.

Carrot
Sweet, Acrid, and Neutral. Enters the liver, lung and spleen channels.
Strengthens the spleen and liver, and downbears Qi.
Treats indigestion, difficulty urinating, dysentery, and cough. Regular consumption can prevent night blindness.

Cauliflower
Sweet, slightly Bitter, slightly Warm. Enters the spleen and stomach channels.
Strengthens the spleen, disperses cold, and relieves pain.
Treats indigestion.

Cayenne Pepper
Acrid and Hot. Enters the spleen and stomach channels.
Dispels cold, fortifies the Stomach, moves Qi and blood, and improves vision.
Treats indigestion and relieves pain.

Celery
Sweet, Bitter and Cool. Enters the bladder, stomach and liver channels.
Clears heat, dispels wind, relieves dampness, disinhibits urination, and relieves
    swelling.
Treats hypertension, headache, dizziness, vertigo, red face and eyes, and blood in
    the urine.

Cherry
Sweet, Aromatic and Warm. Enters the spleen, stomach, lung, heart and kidney
    channels.
Supplements blood and Qi, circulates the Qi and blood, and builds fluids.
Treats weakness, numbness and paralysis of the limbs, low back pain, and
    frostbite.

Chestnut
Sweet and Warm. Enters the spleen, stomach, and kidney channels.
Harmonizes digestion.
Treats upset stomach, diarrhea, weakness in the legs, vomiting blood, nosebleed,
    and blood in the stool.

Chicken
Sweet and Warm. Enters the spleen and stomach channels.
Warms the interior, improves energy.
Treats underweight, poor appetite, diarrhea, edema, frequent urination, vaginal
    discharge and bleeding, scanty lactation, and post-partum weakness.

Chicken Egg
Sweet and Neutral. Enters the spleen, stomach, lung, kidney, and heart
    channels.
Nourishes blood and Yin, brightens eyes, and moistens dryness.
Treats dry cough and dry sore throat, hoarse voice, and blurry vision.

Chicory
Attributes not yet known. Enters the liver and gall bladder channels.

Excites the central nervous system, increases cardiac activity and improves digestion.

Treats indigestion and fatigue.

Chive

Acrid and Warm. Enters the liver, kidney and stomach channels.

Corrects the flow of Qi and blood, harmonizes the stomach, scatters cold, improves appetite, and dissolves blood stasis.

Treats bruises from traumatic injury, nosebleed, blood in the urine, rectal prolapse, indigestion, nausea and vomiting due to cold stomach.

Cinnamon

Acrid, Sweet and Hot. Enters the kidney, spleen and bladder channels.

Warms Yang, warms spleen and stomach, relieves chills, improves blood circulation.

Treats cold limbs, stomach pain, cold-type diarrhea, low back and knee pain, blocked menstruation, post-partum abdominal pain, and numb skin in the elderly. (Note: Avoid this food if you suffer from a heat condition such as fever, blood in the urine or nosebleed, and should not be used by pregnant women.)

Clam

Salty, Sweet and Cold. Enters the spleen, stomach, liver and kidney channels.

Disinhibits urine, saliva and tears, transforms phlegm, softens hard lumps, and strengthens liver and kidney.

Treats goiter, edema, hemorrhoids, pink eye, phlegm, stops dry cough, night sweats, and vaginal discharge.

Clove

Acrid and Warm. Enters the kidney, spleen and stomach channels.

Warms and invigorates Yang.

Treats Stomach cold, vomiting, abdominal pain and diarrhea, clear vaginal discharge, cold uterus infertility, and Yang-deficient impotence.

Coconut

Sweet and Warm. Enters the spleen, stomach, and large intestine channels.

Engenders fluids, disinhibits urination, and expels worms.

Treats thirst after dehydration or diarrhea, tapeworm, diarrhea, and premature aging.

Coffee

Bitter, Acrid and Warm. Enters the lung, liver, kidney, and stomach channels.
Moves the Qi and blood, and disinhibits urination.
Treats chronic bronchitis, emphysema, and alcohol hangover.

Coriander

Acrid and Warm. Enters the lung, stomach and spleen channels.
Facilitates sweating, helps bring out rashes, strengthens and descends stomach
   Qi.
Treats initial stage of measles, and indigestion.

Corn

Sweet and Neutral. Enters the heart, lung, spleen, liver, stomach, gall bladder, and
   bladder channels.
Boosts the lungs, calms the heart, and disinhibits urination.
Treats difficult urination, gallstones, hepatitis, jaundice, and hypertension.

Crab

Salty and Cold. Enters the liver and stomach channels.
Clears heat, moves the blood, and mends bones.
Treats fractures and dislocations, tinea, scabies and can be used topically to treat
   scalding burns.

Crayfish (including lobster)

Sweet, Salty, and Warm. Enters the liver and kidney channels.
Supplements kidneys, and boosts yang.
Treats bone and joint pain.

Cucumber

Sweet and Cool. Enters the spleen, stomach and large intestine channels.
Clears Heat, and replenishes fluids.
Treats pinkeye, burns, thirst and inhibited urination.

Dill

Acrid and Warm. Enters the spleen, kidney and stomach channels.
Warms Yang, dispels cold, moves Qi, relieves food poisoning from fish or beef.
Treats abdominal distention, indigestion, poor appetite, vomiting and low back
   pain.

Duck
Sweet and Level. Enters the lung and kidney channels.
Moistens dryness, nourishes the stomach.
Treats dry cough, irritability, edema, and thirst.

Eel
Sweet and Warm. Enters the liver, spleen and kidney channels.
Strengthens sinews and bones.
Treats pain, urinary block, dysentery, and hemorrhoids.

Eggplant
Sweet and Warm. Enters the large intestine, stomach, and spleen channels.
Clears heat, cools the blood, and promotes bowel movements.
Treats bleeding hemorrhoids, blood in the urine, breast abscesses, swellings, and
   sores.

Fennel
Acrid and Warm. Enters the liver, kidney, spleen, bladder, and stomach
   channels.
Corrects the flow of Qi, harmonizes the stomach.
Treats cold, low back pain, flatulence, abdominal distention, indigestion, poor
   appetite, vomiting, and menstrual pain.

Fig
Sweet and Neutral. Enters the spleen, stomach, and large intestine channels.
Strengthens the spleen, harmonizes the stomach, engenders fluids, and unblocks
   the stool.
Treats indigestion, dry-type constipation, dysentery, hemorrhoids, dry and sore
   throat, and dry cough.

Frog
Sweet and Cool. Enters the bladder, intestines and stomach channels.
Clears heat, resolves toxins, and disperses swelling.
Treats fever, superficial edema, dysentery, and pediatric hot-type sores.

Garlic
Acrid and Warm. Enters the spleen, stomach and lung channels.
Moves stuck Qi, warms the spleen, disperses masses, resolves toxins, and kills
   parasites.

Treats food stagnation, swelling, abdominal distention, diarrhea and dysentery, and whooping cough. Also can prevent and treat the flu.

Ginger (dried)
Acrid and Hot. Enters the spleen, stomach, and lung channels.
Warms the center, dispels cold, and frees the circulation.
Treats heart and abdominal cold-pain, cold limbs, vomiting and diarrhea (cold type), cold-lung panting, and nosebleeds.

Ginger (raw)
Acrid and slightly Warm. Enters the spleen, stomach, and lung channels.
Disperses cold, transforms phlegm and stops vomiting.
Treats the common cold (in the cold-phase), vomiting, asthma, and coughing up phlegm.

Ginseng
Sweet, Slightly Bitter, and Warm. Enters the lung and spleen channels.
Boosts the Qi, calms the spirit, and engenders fluids.
Treats weak cough, fatigue, insomnia, agitation, impotence, frequent urination, digestion, excessive perspiration, diarrhea, diabetes, vaginal bleeding, and poor digestion.

Grape
Sweet, Sour, and Neutral. Enters the lung, spleen and kidney channels.
Supplements Qi and blood, strengthens sinews and bones, and disinhibits urination.
Treats weak cough, heart palpitations, night sweats, urinary difficulties, and edema.

Grapefruit
Sweet, Sour, and Cold. Enters the lung, spleen, and stomach channels.
Corrects the flow of Qi, engenders fluids, and transforms phlegm,
Treats dry cough with phlegm, indigestion, burping, excessive salivation in pregnancy, poor appetite in pregnancy, and alcohol hangover.

Grapefruit Peel (Boil in a tea.)
Acrid, Sweet, Bitter and Warm. Enters the spleen, kidney, and bladder channels.
Corrects the flow of Qi, downbears, transforms phlegm, and eliminates dampness.

Treats nausea and vomiting, abdominal distention and pain, indigestion, and pediatric diarrhea.

Green Bean (string bean)
Sweet and Neutral. Enters the spleen and kidney channels.
Strengthens spleen and kidneys.
Treats diarrhea, diabetes, vomiting, white vaginal discharge, and frequent urination.

Green Onion
Acrid and Warm. Enters the lung and stomach channels.
Induces perspiration.
Treats headache, constipation, retention of urine, abdominal pain and dysentery.

Guava
Sweet, Astringent, and Warm. Enters the lung, spleen, intestines and stomach channels.
Strengthens the spleen, and engenders fluids.
Treats diarrhea and helps hoarse throat.

Hazelnut
Sweet, Aromatic, Slimy, and Neutral. Channels entered not yet known.
Strengthens the spleen, opens the stomach, supplements Qi and blood, brightens the eyes.
Treats diarrhea and fatigue.

Honey
Sweet, Glossy, and Neutral. Enters the lung, spleen, and large intestine channels.
Strengthens the center, moistens dryness, relaxes tension, and resolves toxins.
Treats dry cough in the lung, dry-type constipation, hypertension, heart disease, liver disease, stomach pain, runny nose, mouth sores, and can be used externally to treat burns.

Job's Tears (pearled barley)
Sweet, Bland and slightly Cold. Enters the spleen, lung and kidney channels.
Strengthens the spleen, eliminates damp heat, expels pus, and disinhibits urination.
Treats diarrhea, urinary difficulties, edema, and lung or intestinal abscesses.

Kelp (Don't overlook sea vegetables.)
Salty and Cold. Enters the kidney, liver, lung, and stomach channels.
Softens hardness, transforms phlegm, drains heat and dampness.
Treats goiter, difficulty swallowing, swelling and pain in the testes, vaginal discharge, and edema.

Kidney Bean
Sweet, Bland, and Neutral. Channels entered not yet known.
Promotes urination, reduces edema and swelling.
Treats fluid retention, urinary block, edema and swelling.

Kiwi Fruit
Sweet, Sour and Cool. Enters the spleen and stomach channels.
Clears heat, engenders fluids, and strengthens the spleen.
Treats diarrhea, sore throat with fever, jaundice, red and painful urination, indigestion, and loss of appetite.

Kohlrabi
Bitter and Neutral. Channels entered not yet known.
Detoxifies.
Treats indigestion, jaundice, diabetes, alcoholism, and nosebleed.

Kumquat
Acrid, Sweet, slightly Sour, and Warm. Enters the liver, spleen, kidney, and stomach channels.
Corrects the flow of Qi, harmonizes the stomach, dries dampness and transforms phlegm.
Treats abdominal distention and pain, nausea, hypertension, indigestion, and cough with clear, thin phlegm, and resolves masses.

Lamb
Sweet and Warm. Enters the spleen and kidney channels.
Boosts the Qi, warms the center.
Treats low back pain, knee pain and weakness, postpartum chill, underweight, and abdominal pain.

Leek
Acrid and Warm. Enters the liver and lung channels.
Boosts the Qi and Yang, moves the blood, and expels cold.

Treats stomach fire and difficulty swallowing.

Lemon
Sour, Astringent, and Warm. Enters the lung, spleen and stomach channels.
Transforms phlegm, stops cough, engenders fluids, and strengthens the spleen.
Treats thirst, dry and painful throat, indigestion, diabetes, and cough with phlegm.

Lettuce (Eat several different types.)
Bitter, Sweet, and Cool. Enters the stomach and large intestine channels.
Clears heat, disinhibits urine, and promotes lactation.
Treats urinary difficulties (including blood) and poor lactation.

Licorice
Sweet and Neutral. Enters the spleen, stomach, and lung channels.
Harmonizes the actions of foods and herbs, and lubricates the lungs.
Treats constipation, abdominal pain, fatigue, cough, convulsions, sore throat, digestive ulcers, and toxicity from drug or food poisoning.

Lichee Fruit
Sweet, slightly Sour, and Warm. Enters the liver, spleen and stomach channels.
Engenders fluids and supplements blood, corrects the flow of Qi, and stops pain.
Treats thirst, Qi-deficiency, diarrhea, stomach ache, hiccups, asthma, and hernia pain.

Longan Fruit
Sweet and Warm. Enters the heart and spleen channels.
Nourishes heart and spleen.
Treats insomnia, palpitations, poor memory, restlessness, and blurry vision.

Loquat Fruit
Sweet, Sour and Cool. Enters the lung, spleen and stomach channels.
Clears heat, moistens the lungs, stops thirst, and directs Qi downward.
Treats dry and sore throat, and dry cough.

Lotus Root and Seed
Sweet and Cool (slightly Warm when cooked). Enters the heart, spleen, and stomach channels.

Clears heat, cools the blood, stops bleeding, and disperses stasis.
Treats diarrhea, nosebleeds, coughing blood, vaginal discharge and bleeding, and urinary heat.

Malt

Sweet and slightly Warm. Enters the spleen and stomach channels.
Promotes digestion, and moves downward.
Treats indigestion, abdominal distention, vomiting, diarrhea, poor appetite, and breast swelling.

Maltose

Sweet and Warm. Enters the spleen, stomach, and lung channels.
Produces fluids and lubricates dryness.
Treats fatigue, abdominal pain, thirst, constipation, vomiting of blood, dry throat and dry cough.

Mango

Sweet, Sour and Cool. Enters the lung, spleen, and stomach channels.
Corrects the flow of Qi, strengthens the spleen and stomach.
Treats cough, panting, wheezing, bleeding gums, vomiting and indigestion.

Marjoram

Acrid and Cool. Enters the lung, spleen, and stomach channels.
Disinhibits urination, opens the stomach.
Treats heatstroke, edema, and food stagnation.

Milk (human)

Sweet, Salty, and Level. Enters the lung, spleen, heart, kidney, liver, and stomach channels.
Supplements blood, builds muscle and bones, strengthens stomach and spleen, sharpens hearing and brightens the eyes.

Milk (cow)

Sweet and Neutral. Enters the heart, lung, and stomach channels.
Boosts the lung and stomach, engenders fluids, and moistens intestines.
Treats difficulty in swallowing, weakness and dry-type constipation.

Milk (goat)

Sweet and Warm. Enters the lung, kidney and stomach channels.

Warms and moistens. Supplements lung and kidney Qi, and harmonizes small
intestine.

Treats emaciation and thirst, burping, and mouth sores.

Millet

Sweet, Salty and Cool. Enters the kidney, spleen and stomach channels.
Harmonizes the stomach, boosts the kidney, eliminates heat and resolves toxins.
Treats vomiting, thirst, and diarrhea.

Molasses

Sweet and Warm. Enters the lung, spleen, and stomach channels.
Strengthens the spleen, boost the Qi, moistens the lung and engenders fluids.
Treats abdominal distention and dry-type cough.

Mulberry

Sweet, Sour and Cool. Enters the lung, spleen, liver, and kidney channels.
Stops cough, disinhibits urination, disperses swelling, supplements the kidneys
and liver, brightens the eyes and nourishes the blood.
Treats blurry vision, night blindness, dizziness, tinnitus, premature graying hair,
and thirst.

Mung bean

Sweet and Cool. Enters the heart and stomach channels.
Clears heat, resolves toxins and disperses summer-heat.
Treats heatstroke, water swelling, dysentery and diarrhea, abscesses, and medicinal
toxicity.

Muskmelon

Sweet and Cold. Enters the heart and stomach channels.
Reduces fever, quenches thirst and promotes urination.
Treats cough, constipation, liver disease, and difficulty urinating.

Mushroom (button)

Sweet and Cool. Enters the intestines, stomach and lung channels.
Opens the stomach, corrects the flow of Qi, transforms phlegm, quiets the spirit,
resolves toxins, and expresses rashes.
Treats vomiting, diarrhea, fatigue and weakness, dry mouth, cough with phlegm,
and oppression in the chest.

Mushroom (oyster)
Sweet and Slightly Warm. Enters the spleen, stomach, and liver channels.
Strengthens the spleen, relieves spasms, and eliminates dampness.
Treats poor appetite and pain.

Mushroom (shiitake)
Sweet and Neutral. Enters the stomach channels.
Prevents rickets, anemia, and measles.
Treats cough, fish poisoning, and blood in the urine.

Mussel
Salty and Warm. Enters the liver and kidney channels.
Supplements the kidney and invigorates Yang, nourishes the liver, strengthens the
    sinews, moistens dryness and replenishes essence.
Treats goiter, dizziness, vertigo, night sweats, low back pain, vaginal bleeding and
    vaginal discharge, impotence, and vomiting of blood.

Mustard Greens
Acrid and Warm. Enters the lung and stomach channels.
Warms, transforms and expels phlegm, scatters cold, corrects the flow of Qi and
    blood, and warms the center. Regulates respiration.
Treats cold phlegm, cough and panting with profuse white phlegm, and chest
    oppression.

Nutmeg
Acrid and Warm. Enters the large intestine, stomach, and spleen channels.
Stops diarrhea and secures the intestines. Warms the center and moves the Qi.
Treats abdominal pain and swelling, vomiting, and diarrhea.

Oats
Sweet and Neutral. Enters the spleen, stomach, lung, and large intestine channels.
Strengthens the spleen, boosts the Qi, and moistens dryness.
Treats spontaneous perspiration and dry bowels.

Olive
Sweet, Sour, Astringent, and Neutral. Enters the lung and stomach channels.
Astringes and secures fluids, engenders fluids, and moistens the lung.
Treats dry throat, dry cough, coughing up blood, enduring diarrhea, and alcohol
    hangover.

Onion

Acrid and Warm. Enters the lung, stomach, spleen, liver and large intestine channels.

Warms the interior, scatters cold, dispels wind, moves the Qi and blood, and resolves masses.

Treats common cold (in the cold-phase), diarrhea, and worms.

Orange

Sweet, Sour, and Cool. Enters the lung, bladder, and stomach channels.

Opens the stomach, corrects the flow of Qi, induces urination, stops thirst, and moistens the lung.

Treats chest constriction, vomiting, poor appetite, dry cough, and dry-lung cough.

Orange Peel (Brew in a tea or add to stir-fry.)

Sour, Bitter, Aromatic, and Warm. Enters the lung, spleen, and stomach channels.

Corrects the flow of Qi, harmonizes the center and loosens the diaphragm, dries dampness and transforms phlegm.

Treats indigestion, abdominal distention and pain, burping, nausea, vomiting, cough with phlegm, and lack of appetite.

Oyster

Salty, Sweet, and Neutral. Enters the liver and kidney channels.

Supplements the kidney and liver.

Treats goiter, night sweats, stress, nervousness, vaginal discharge, insomnia, restlessness, and agitation.

Papaya

Sweet and Cold. Enters the spleen and stomach channels.

Fortifies the spleen and stomach, and resolves thirst.

Treats heat stroke, difficulty in bowel movements, fever with thirst, indigestion, scanty lactation, and persistent cough.

Pea

Sweet and Level. Enters the heart, spleen, stomach and large intestine channels.

Fortifies the spleen, disinhibits urination, moistens the intestines and frees the stool.

Treats indigestion, edema, and dry-type constipation.

Peach

Sweet, Sour, and Warm. Enters the stomach and intestine channels.

Engenders fluids, moistens the intestines, moves the blood and disperses nodules and swelling,

Treats thirst and dry-type constipation, cough, and excessive perspiration.

Peanut

Sweet and Neutral. Enters the spleen and lung channels.

Moistens the lung, harmonizes the stomach, and stops bleeding.

Treats dry cough, nausea, and scanty lactation.

Pear

Sweet, Slightly Sour, and Cool. Enters the lung and stomach channels.

Engenders fluids, moistens dryness, clears heat, and transforms phlegm.

Treats heat cough, phlegm cough, constipation, mania, difficulty swallowing, and constipation.

Peppermint

Acrid and Cool. Enters the lung and liver channels.

Clears heat, clears the head and the eyes, disinhibits the throat, expresses rashes, and corrects the flow of Qi,

Treats common cold (in the warm phase), fever, headache, cough, sore throat, red eyes, abdominal and side distention, irritability, canker sores, premenstrual breast tenderness and abdominal distention.

Persimmon

Sweet, Astringent, and Cold. Enters the spleen, lung, and stomach channels.

Moistens the lung, engenders fluids, and strengthens the spleen.

Treats epigastric pain, cough and wheeze, diarrhea and dysentery, bleeding hemorrhoids, hypertension, mouth sores, dry and painful throat, hiccups, coughing blood, and blood in the urine.

Pineapple

Sweet, slightly Astringent, and Neutral. Channels entered not yet known.

Supplements the spleen, engenders fluids, and promotes urination.

Treats indigestion, vomiting, abdominal distention, low blood pressure, weakness in the hands and feet, fever with thirst, edema, vomiting, and difficulty urinating.

Pine Nut

Sweet and Warm. Enters the liver, lung and large intestine channels.

Nourishes fluids, extinguishes wind, moistens the lung and large intestine.

Treats constipation, dizziness, dry cough or coughing up blood.

Plum

Bitter, Sour, Astringent, and Cool. Enters the spleen, stomach, and bladder channels.

Clears heat, disinhibits urine, and promotes digestion.

Treats indigestion, bleeding gums, liver disease, gingivitis, chronic sore throat, and sores in the mouth or on the tongue.

Pomegranate

Bitter, Sour, Astringent, and Cool. Enters the lung, spleen, and stomach channels.

Clears heat, moistens the lung, and stops cough.

Treats dry and sore throat, hoarse voice, enduring cough, diarrhea and dysentery, and red, weepy skin abscesses.

Pork

Sweet, Salty and Neutral. Enters the spleen, stomach, and kidney channels.

Supplements the kidneys, nourishes the blood, enriches Yin, and moistens dryness.

Treats heat damaging fluids, underweight, weakness, post-partum blood deficiency, dry cough and dry-type constipation.

Potato

Sweet and Neutral. Enters the spleen and Stomach channels.

Boosts the Qi, strengthens the spleen, clears heat, and relieves spasms.

Treats hepatitis, breast abscesses, laryngitis, tonsilitis, mumps, lack of energy, burns, and ulcers in the stomach or intestines.

Pumpkin (and winter squash)

Sweet and Warm. Enters the spleen and stomach channels.

Boosts the center, supplements Qi, resolves toxins and dissolves phlegm.

Treats inflammation, pain, bronchial asthma, edema, vomiting blood, and intestinal worms.

Pumpkin Seed

Sweet and Warm. Enters the spleen, stomach, and large intestine channels.

Kills worms, moistens the intestines and frees the stool.

Treats parasites, bleeding hemorrhoids, and insufficient lactation.

Radish

Acrid, Sweet and Cool. Enters the lung and stomach channels.

Disperses accumulations and stagnations, resolves toxins, and descends the Qi.

Treats food stagnation, cough with phlegm, coughing blood, nosebleed, dysentery, thirst, and migraine headache.

Raspberry

Sour, Sweet, and Warm. Enters the liver and kidney channels.

Nourishes liver and kidneys.

Treats frequent urination and warms the womb.

Red Date

Sweet and Neutral. Enters the spleen and stomach channels.

Supplements the spleen, boosts the Qi, nourishes the blood and calms the spirit.

Treats blood and Qi deficiency, fatigue, shortness of breath, poor appetite, loose stools, irritability, restlessness, and nervousness.

Rice

Sweet and Neutral. Enters the spleen and stomach channels.

Supplements the center and the spleen, boosts the Qi and harmonizes the stomach.

Treats excessive thirst, diarrhea, and dysentery.

Rice (Glutinous)

Sweet and Warm. Enters the lung, spleen and stomach channels.

Supplements the lungs, fortifies the spleen.

Treats diarrhea and spontaneous perspiration.

Rice (wild)

Sweet and Cool. Enters the stomach, bladder, and large intestine channels.

Clears heat, engenders fluids, promotes urination, drains dampness, and promotes bowel movement.

Treats constipation, urinary block, and dryness.

Rice Bran

Sweet, Acrid, and Neutral. Enters the stomach and large intestine channels.

Directs Qi downward.

Treats difficulty swallowing, and beriberi.

Rosemary

Acrid and Warm. Enters the lung and stomach channels.

Scatters cold, moves the Qi, and opens the stomach.

Treats common cold (in the cold-phase), headache, abdominal pain, indigestion, and menstrual pain.

Royal Jelly

Attributes and channels entered not yet known. Promotes growth and inhibits aging.

Treats slow development, loss of weight, poor appetite, hepatitis, rheumatoid arthritis, anemia and gastric ulcers.

Saffron

Sweet and Neutral. Enters the heart and liver channels.

Moves blood, resolves stasis, and stops pain.

Treats blocked menstruation, painful menstruation, postpartum dizziness, heart and chest pain, traumatic injury, vomiting blood, and post-partum abdominal pain.

Salt

Salty and Cold. Enters the stomach, kidney, large intestine, and small intestine channels.

Induces vomiting, disperses phlegm, resolves toxins, and clears fire.

Treats blocked urine or stool, phlegm in the chest, bleeding gums, sore throat, toothache, cataracts, and insect and snake bites.

Scallions

Acrid and Warm. Enters the lung and stomach channels.

Warms the Yang, and resolves toxins.

Treats cold and chills, headache, cold abdominal pain, blocked urine or stool, dysentery, and worms.

Seaweed

Salty and Cold. Channels entered not yet known.

Softens hardness, eliminates phlegm, disinhibits urination, and clears heat.

Treats hard masses, difficulty urinating, beriberi, and goiter.

Sesame Seed
Sweet and Neutral. Enters the liver and kidney channels.
Supplements the liver and kidneys, and moistens the interior.
Treats vertigo, paralysis, premature graying of the hair, and insufficient lactation.

Sesame Oil
Sweet and Cool. Channels entered not yet known.
Detoxifies, moistens dryness, promotes bowel movements, and produces muscles.
Treats constipation, ulcers, cracked skin, and scabies.

Shark
Sweet, Salty, and Neutral. Channels entered not yet known.
Boosts the Qi and opens the stomach.
Treats weakness.

Shrimp
Sweet and Warm. Enters the liver and kidney channels.
Nourishes the liver and kidneys.
Treats impotence and insufficient lactation.

Sichuan Pepper
Acrid, Hot, and slightly toxic. Enters the kidney, spleen, and stomach channels.
Warms the center and strengthens the spleen, scatters cold, kills worms, and stops
    pain.
Treats cold abdominal pain, vomiting, diarrhea, and worms.

Sorghum
Sweet and Warm. Enters the spleen and stomach channels.
Warms the center, fortifies the spleen, and dries dampness.
Treats indigestion, inhibited urination, and dysentery.

Soybean (black)
Sweet and Neutral. Enters the spleen and large intestine channels.
Moves the blood, and resolves toxins.
Treats water retention, distention, jaundice, edema, tight joints, muscle cramps,
    lockjaw, swelling, and drug poisoning.

Soybean (yellow)
Sweet and Neutral. Enters the spleen and large intestine channels.

Strengthens the spleen, loosens the intestines, moistens dryness and expels water.

Treats diarrhea, dysentery, abdominal distention, toxemia in pregnancy, sores, and bleeding due to traumatic injury.

Soybean Sprout
Sweet and Cool. Enters the spleen, stomach, and large intestine channels.

Clears heat, disinhibits urination, and harmonizes the Stomach.

Treats food stagnation, hot stomach, edema, and improves male fertility (sprouts have a motile nature).

Soy Sauce
Salty and Cold. Enters the spleen, stomach, and kidney channels.

Eliminates heat, and resolves toxins.

Treats bee/wasp stings and burns (applied topically).

Spearmint
Acrid and Warm. Enters the lung, liver and stomach channels.

Scatters cold, moves the Qi, and stops pain.

Treats indigestion, abdominal pain, common cold (cold phase), headache, and menstrual pain.

Spinach
Sweet and Cool. Enters the liver, large intestine and stomach channels.

Nourishes the blood, stops bleeding, and moistens dryness.

Treats nosebleeds, alcoholism, thirst, blood in the stool, and constipation. Improves vision.

Squash (summer squash)
Sweet and Cold. Enters the spleen, stomach, and large intestine channels.

Clears heat, opens the waterways, resolves toxins, relieves inflammation, relieves thirst, and calms agitation.

Treats urinary difficulty, edema, heat stroke, roundworms, and irritability.

Squid
Salty, Sweet, and Neutral. Enters the liver and kidney channels.

Nourishes liver and kidneys.

Treats vaginal bleeding or discharge, amenorrhea, and blood deficiency.

Star Fruit
Sweet, Sour, and Cool. Channels entered not yet known.
Reduces fever, produces fluids, promotes urination, and detoxifies.
Treats cough and fever, toothache, kidney or bladder stones, indigestion, canker sores, and alcohol hangover.

Strawberry
Sweet, Sour, and Cool. Enters the lung, spleen, liver, kidney, and stomach channels.
Engenders fluids, moistens the lungs, nourishes liver and kidneys.
Treats dry cough, thirst, sore or swollen throat, indigestion, frequent urination, alcohol hangover, dizziness and weakness after a long illness.

Sugar (brown)
Sweet and Warm. Enters the liver, spleen, and stomach channels.
Supplements the spleen, moves the blood, and transforms stasis.
Treats abdominal pain, dysentery, and abdominal pain after retention of placenta.

Sugar (white)
Sweet and Neutral. Enters the lung and spleen channels.
Supplements the center and boosts the Qi, harmonizes the stomach, and moistens the lungs.
Treats dry lungs, common cold (cold-phase), coughing and panting, stomach ache, mouth sores and toothache.

Sugar Cane
Sweet and Cold. Enters the lungs and stomach channels.
Lubricates dryness, promotes urination, directs Qi downward, and produces fluids.
Treats vomiting, dry cough, and constipation.

Sunflower Seed
Sweet and Neutral. Channels entered not yet known.
Strengthens the spleen, and moistens the intestines.
Treats dry constipation, and dysentery with pus or blood.

Sweet Potato
Sweet and Neutral or Cool. Enters the large intestine, stomach and spleen channels.

Strengthens the spleen, boosts the Qi, enriches kidneys, and engenders fluids.
Treats thirst, diarrhea, constipation, weak kidneys, and premature ejaculation.

Tangerine
Sweet, Sour and Neutral. Enters the lung and stomach channels.

Engenders fluids, quenches thirst, promotes appetite, dissolves phlegm, moistens
 the lung and descends counterflow Qi.

Treats thirst, vomiting, loss of appetite, chest congestion, and cough with profuse
 phlegm.

Taro Root
Acrid, Sweet, and Neutral. Enters the stomach and large intestine channels.

Strengthens the spleen and stomach and dissolves masses.

Treats loss of appetite. Use topically for inflammation, swelling and pain.

Tea (Green) (The greatest beverage in the world).
Bitter, Sweet, and Cool. Enters the lung, heart, and stomach channels.

Clears the head and eyes, transforms phlegm, moves food, disinhibits urination,
 and resolves toxins.

Treats headache, dizziness, excessive sleeping, cloudy thinking, thirst, food
 stagnation, and dysentery. Increases metabolism, decreases appetite, and
 prevents: cancer, heart disease, vascular disease, and dental cavities. Regulates
 blood pressure and blood sugar, lowers lipids, triglycerides, and cholesterol.
 Reduces pain, improves mood, strengthens bones, and prevents chromosomal
 degradation in the eggs and sperm.

Thyme
Acrid and Warm. Enters the lung and stomach channels.

Dispels cold, moves the Qi, opens the stomach, downbears upwardly rebellious
 Qi, and stops cough.

Treats common cold (cold phase) with headache, cough, body aches, sore throat,
 whooping cough, bronchitis, laryngitis, nausea, vomiting, indigestion, and
 abdominal distention.

Tobacco
Acrid, Toxic, and Warm. Channels entered not yet known.

Moves the Qi, relieves pain, dries dampness, and warms cold.

Treats indigestion, abdominal distention, headache, and arthritis.

Tofu

Sweet and cool. Enters the spleen, stomach, and large intestine channels.

Boosts the Qi, harmonizes the stomach, engenders fluids, moistens dryness, clears heat, and resolves toxins.

Treats red eyes, diabetes, sulfur poisoning, and recurrent dysentery.

Tomato

Sweet, Sour, and Slightly Cold. Enters the stomach channel.

Clears heat, moistens dryness, stops thirst, opens the stomach, disperses accumulations, moves the blood, and transforms stasis.

Treats oral sores, red eyes, dizziness, hypertension, constipation, and indigestion due to over-eating.

Turmeric

Acrid, Bitter and Warm. Enters the spleen, stomach, and liver channels.

Moves the blood, frees the menses, moves the Qi and stops pain.

Treats blocked menstruation (amenorrhea), painful menstruation, pain and swelling due to traumatic injury, and abdominal pain.

Turnip

Acrid, Sweet, Bitter and Cool. Enters the spleen, stomach, and lung channels.

Clears heat, eliminates dampness, transforms phlegm, moves stagnation, promotes digestion, and resolves toxins.

Treats breast abscesses, phlegm, heat cough, food stagnation with heat, and spastic urination.

Venison

Sweet and Warm. Enters the liver and kidney channels.

Nourishes the liver and invigorates the kidneys, strengthens the bones and sinews.

Treats low back pain, knee soreness and weakness, premature ejaculation, impotence, and male infertility.

Vinegar

Sour, Bitter and Warm. Enters the liver and stomach channels.

Scatters stasis, stops bleeding, resolves toxins, and kills worms.

Treats post-partum dizziness, jaundice, coughing blood, vomiting blood, blood in the stool, nosebleeds, vaginal itching, and poisoning from fish, meat, or vegetables.

Walnut

Sweet and Warm. Enters the kidney and lung channels. .

Supplements the kidneys, warms the lung, moistens the intestines, and frees the stool.

Treats panting, coughing, wheezing, low back pain, lower leg weakness, impotence, frequent urination, kidney stones, and dry constipation.

Water Chestnut

Sweet, Bland, and Cool. Enters the lung, spleen, stomach, bladder, and large intestine channels.

Clears heat, and transforms phlegm. Engenders fluids, disinhibits urination, and lowers blood pressure.

Treats lung heat with sticky phlegm, fever with thirst, dry and painful throat, red, scanty or painful urination, red and painful eyes, measles, dysentery with blood in the stool, bleeding hemorrhoids, diabetes, and hypertension.

Watercress

Acrid, Bitter and Cool. Enters the lung, stomach and bladder channels.

Clears heat, stops thirst, moistens the lung, and disinhibits urination.

Treats thirst, restlessness, irritability, dry and sore throat, and cough with yellow phlegm.

Watermelon

Sweet and Cold. Enters the heart, stomach, and bladder channels.

Clears heat and heatstroke, stops thirst, and disinhibits urination.

Treats heatstroke, thirst, inhibited urination, sore throat, and oral sores.

Wheat

Sweet and Cool. Enters the heart, spleen, and kidney channels.

Nourishes the heart and kidneys, eliminates heat, and stops thirst,

Treats heat and thirst, diarrhea, dysentery, swellings, and bleeding due to traumatic injury.

Yam

Sweet and Neutral. Enters the lung, spleen, and kidney channels.

Strengthens the lung and spleen.

Treats chronic diarrhea, cough, diabetes, vaginal discharge, and frequent urination.

Yogurt

Sweet, Sour, and Warm. Enters the lung, liver, stomach, and large intestine channels.

Moistens the lung and large intestines, and resolves thirst.

Treats dry cough and dry constipation.

Chapter Twenty

Recipes

This is not a cookbook, but these recipes incorporate the concepts of the Asian Diet. If you would like to contribute a recipe that you think adheres to the principles, please visit www.theasiandiet.com to submit it, but first:

Tips for making rice

Everybody should buy a rice cooker/warmer (it is better if you can find one with a cast-iron or stainless steel bowl, (avoid aluminum), make sure it has a locking lid). Cooking rice on a stove is not that difficult, but I find it to be a chore. I have to keep my mind on it and an eye on it; and it takes nearly an hour. My wife is Korean and I converted when we got married, so I am now also Asian. That means we have rice almost every day. With a rice cooker/warmer, you put in 2 cups of rice, three cups of water, close the lid and press Start. Then you come back in an hour, or come back in 10 hours. The rice is hot, fresh and good to go. Close the lid, go to bed, and go to work the next day, come home . . . the rice is still hot, still fresh, and still good-to-go. It will stay hot and fresh for 3 days as long as you fluff the rice at least once a day. Fresher is better if you have the time, but this is a way to have good food on hand at all times. Instant rice is not good, nor is the boil-in-plastic-bags brand. Just get a rice cooker. Trust me, it's so easy you'll love it.

Brown rice and other grains have a longer cooking time than white rice, unless they are soaked first. So once a month we buy a bag of mixed grains from our local health food store or Asian market. It will have some barley, some brown and long grain rice, maybe some millet, wheat, beans, etc. Then we soak the grain in a bowl of filtered water overnight. In the morning, we pour off the water and put the mix in one-cup portions into baggies and freeze them. Then, when we want to make rice, we will use two cups of white rice and one cup of the mix. This way we get a wide variety of grains, but cut the concentration of the harder-to-digest grains with the white rice. Rice should be rinsed a few times in filtered water before cooking it.

Stir Fry (for four)

Use 8 ounces of chicken, crab, shrimp, beef or pork. Brown the meat in a skillet with a little bit of oil (mix it up: olive, vegetable, palm, etc.). Add some of any or all of the following, chopped into bite-sized pieces:

* Bok Choy
* Pea Pods
* Broccoli
* Carrots
* Scallions
* Onions
* Mushrooms
* Water chestnuts
* Kale
* Peppers (Green, Red, Yellow, Purple, Jalepeno, etc)
* Garlic (minced)
* Ginger (minced)
* Jicama
* Spinach
* Mustard Greens
* Collard Greens
* Peanuts
* Beans (Green, Soy, Navy, Wax, Lima, etc)
* Almonds
* Walnuts
* Cabbage – Napa, Head, Red
* Zucchini (Courgette)
* Squash
* Celery
* Fiddlehead Greens
* Turnip
* Cauliflower
* Asparagus
* Bamboo Shoots
* Wax Beans
* Eggplant
* Okra
* Fennel

* Corn
* Potato

Add the chopped ingredients and stir-fry with the protein and add 1 tub of organic tofu, cubed. Add a little soy, teriyaki, or fish sauce, salt or pepper. Serve with rice or add cooked noodles (buckwheat, wheat, rice, wild rice, bean-thread) to the last few minutes of stirring. There are so many variations that can be made from this theme; so there is no chance to get bored with it.

Bi Bim Bop

Ingredients

* 8-16 oz beef steak or tofu
* 3/4 cup sesame sauce
* 1/2 pound bean sprouts (soy or mung bean)
* 3/4 ounces fresh spinach
* 2 tsp. black pepper
* 1 tsp. salt
* 1 tsp. vinegar
* 1 daikon radish or turnip
* 2 cucumbers
* 3/4 cup raw sugar, stevia, or agave nectar
* 4 eggs
* 1/2 cup rice wine
* Any additional vegetables of your choice
* 1 cup red pepper paste sauce (if available)

Prepare the Beef Marinade:
Combine and whisk a half-cup of soy sauce, sesame oil, sweetener, rice wine, and 1 teaspoon of black pepper in a bowl.

Prepare the Beef:
The beef should be sliced paper-thin. Marinate the beef for at about 3 hours or even overnight. Brown the meat in a large skillet with a tablespoon of oil over medium heat, and then remove from heat.
Fry or scramble the Eggs

Prepare the Vegetables:
Chop off the stalks from the bunch of spinach. Peel the cucumbers, split them in half and de-seed them with a spoon, julienne them into long, thin strips. Peel and julienne the radish. Many other vegetables can also be added, such as: fiddlehead greens, scallions, carrots, turnip, kelp, kim chee, perilla, lettuce, cabbage, bok choy, broccoli, yam, sweet potato stem, etc.

Blanch the Vegetables:
Boil a pot of water. Into the boiling water place the bean sprouts and wait until the water boils again, then remove them with a slotted spoon. Into the same water, drop your spinach leaves and cook them for 20 seconds. Place the

spinach and bean sprouts into a bowl and rinse them with cold water to stop the cooking.

Marinate the Vegetables:
In a small bowl, mix together vegetable sauce: 1/4 cup soy sauce, 1/2 cup sesame oil, 1 teaspoon each of salt and black pepper. Whisk everything together and pour half of the sauce into your bowl of sprouts, the second half into your bowl with spinach, and set them aside. Next, make a vinegar marinade by mixing together remaining sugar, salt, and vinegar. Pour some into the bowl of cucumber strips and some into the bowl of radish strips.

To Serve:
Arrange beef, sprouts, spinach, cucumber, radish and other vegetables over a bowl of rice (white, brown, or mixed). Top off with the fried or scrambled egg and some spicy red pepper sauce (sometimes make it less spicy). Then mix it all up in the bowl and eat it.

The reason this meal is good is that all the veggies are only slightly cooked and the dish has a wide variety of vegetables with not too much of any one thing.

This is the traditional way to make Bi Bim Bop, but sometimes I will just throw lettuce and other chopped veggies into a bowl of hot rice and stir it with some sauce. The heat from the rice cooks the veggies and makes for a quick and healthy meal.

Epilogue

Now you have the tools to change your diet and change your life and while the principles are simple, it may take some practice to incorporate them. This is not an all-or-nothing proposition, so just try to get a little better each week. Not only is this change possible, it is necessary, for you **will** reap the benefits of a longer, healthier and happier life. But remember, food changes take a long time to take effect. Don't get discouraged if you do not notice improvement right away; you should at least notice that things are not getting worse. First we have to stop the nosedive, and then the changes will be for the better. Remember the words of Hippocrates "Let your food be your medicine and let your medicine be your food."

Eat well and you will be well. And that is my wish for all of you. Be well.

Supplemental Information

If you would like to learn more, please read the following books:

Healing with Whole Foods: Asian Traditions and Modern Nutrition by Paul Pitchford

The Tao of Healthy Eating by Bob Flaws

Skinny Bitch by Rory Freedman and Kim Barnouin

In Defense of Food: An Eater's Manifesto by Michael Pollan

Our Stolen Future by Theo Colborn, Diane Dumanoski, and John Peterson Meyers

Chinese Nutrition Therapy: Dietetics in Traditional Chinese Medicine by Joerg Kastner and Anika Moje

Chinese Dietary Therapy by Liu Jilin and George C. Peck

The *Tao Te Ching* (many translations available)

Chinese System of Food Cures: Prevention & Remedies by Henry C. Lu (currently out of print)

Suggestions for Bone Health,
by Dr. HingHau Tsang

Dietary Guidelines

1) Eat plenty of fresh, green vegetables and whole grains. Leafy dark green vegetables – beans, broccoli, sesame seeds, oats, and tofu – are especially rich sources of calcium and magnesium [and] should be a regular part of your diet. Eat foods high in flavonoids, which help stabilize collagen structures, such as blueberries, raspberries and hawthorne berries. Lower protein vegetarian diets are associated with significantly higher bone mineral density – not to mention improved overall health. Trace minerals are also important in helping your body absorb calcium. Eating plenty of green leafy vegetables gives you calcium along with these helpful trace minerals. Boron and manganese are especially important. Foods that contain boron include apples, legumes, almonds, pears and green, leafy vegetables. Foods that include manganese include ginger, buckwheat and oats. The organic matter in our bones consists mainly of collagen, the "glue" that holds together skin, ligaments, tendons and bones. Zinc, copper, beta-carotene and vitamin C are all important to the formation and maintenance of collagen in the body.

2) Avoid soda pop and carbonated beverages and [a] high protein diet. One of the leading contributors to osteoporosis in the U.S. is carbonated soft drinks containing phosphorous. Research has shown a direct link between too much phosphorous and calcium loss. Our other source of excessive phosphorous in the U.S. is eating too much meat. Keep meat consumption to no more than once a day.

3) Avoid caffeine, alcohol, and cigarette smoking. Each of these substances creates a negative calcium balance in the body. Substances called phytates and oxylates bind with calcium in the large intestine and form insoluble salts, rendering the calcium useless. The bone mineral content of smokers is 15-30% lower in women and 10-20% lower in men. Cigarette smoking is a significant risk factor for osteoporosis. Twice as many women with osteoporosis smoke as compared with women who do not have osteoporosis. So no more than one cup of coffee and one alcohol drink per day. If you

---

are at a high risk, I advise elimination. You should also restrict your consumption of refined sugar, sugary drinks and salt. All of these promote calcium loss. For a healthy beverage, drink green tea. Famous for its cancer-fighting properties, green tea is also a good source of vitamin K, which improves bone mineralization.

4) Avoid dairy products. Milk and other dairy products are not the best source of dietary calcium. That's because milk, cheese, and all animal products are high in protein. The more protein you eat, the more calcium you need to neutralize the acidic byproducts of protein. Don't depend on milk to get your calcium. Milk has a poor calcium to magnesium ratio. Your body needs a certain amount of magnesium in order to get the calcium into your bones -- without magnesium, calcium can't build strong bones. In fact, magnesium deficiency may be more common in women with osteoporosis than calcium deficiency.

5) Decrease your sodium intake. Avoid salty processed foods and fast food. Don't salt your food before tasting it.

Exercise your way to stronger bones

Stress or strain on bones stimulates the formation of new bone. Weight-bearing exercise is the only thing besides progesterone found to actually increase bone density in older women. 30 minutes of weight bearing exercise 4-5 times a week. Brisk walking with hand-held weights counts as weight-bearing exercise. Those women who don't exercise continue to lose bone, regardless of what else they are doing. Exercise can help increase flexibility, strength, and coordination as well. A weight lifting program of just half an hour three to four times a week can significantly improve bone density.

AVOID:

1) Antacids with aluminum and don't use aluminum cooking pots.
It has been shown that small amounts of aluminum-containing antacids increase the urinary and fecal excretion of calcium, inhibit absorption of fluoride, and inhibit absorption of phosphorus, creating a negative calcium balance. The calcium is excreted instead of being utilized.

2) H2 blockers such as Tagamet, Zantac and Pepcid.
As we age, we tend to produce less stomach acid. To be absorbed, calcium requires vitamin D and stomach acid. For this reason, it's important to avoid antacids and the H2 blockers, which block or suppress the secretion of stomach acid.

3) Diuretics

Diuretics cause water loss in the body. Along with the water you lose minerals, most notably calcium, magnesium and potassium. They are commonly used to treat high blood pressure, swelling of the lower leg, and congestive heart failure. People who use diuretics have a higher risk of fracture. If you need to use a diuretic, try a gentle herbal one such as dandelion root.

4) Fluoride

There is good, solid scientific evidence that fluoridated drinking water increases your risk of hip fractures by 20-40%. So much fluoride has been put into our water and toothpaste over the past 30 years that levels in our water, food and drink are very high. While eating a normal diet, the average person exceeds the recommended dose. There is also evidence that ingesting high levels of fluoride can cause abnormal bone growth. Please avoid fluoride in all forms, including toothpastes and mouthwashes. If you are at a high risk for osteoporosis, I recommend a water filter that removes fluoride.

5) High Dose of Cortisone

A well-known risk for osteoporosis is long-term treatment with the synthetic cortisones such as Prednisone. While progesterone gives bones the message to grow, the cortisones give bones the message to stop growing. If you must be on a cortisone, talk to your doctor about using a low dose natural cortisone called hydrocortisone rather than the synthetic cortisones.

Reference

1. Heaney RP, Nordin BEC. Calcium effects on phosphorus absorption: implications for the prevention and co-therapy of osteoporosis. J Am Coll Nutr 2002;21:239-44.
2. Mannan MT, Tucker K, Dawson-Hughes B, et al. Effect of dietary protein on bone loss in elderly men and women: the Framingham Osteoporosis Study. J Bone Mineral Res 2000;15:2504-12.
3. Espauella J, Guyer H, Diaz-Escriu F, et al. Nutritional supplementation of elderly hip fracture patients. A randomized, double-blind placebo-controlled trial. Age Ageing 2000;29:425-31.
4. Sahota O. Osteoporosis and the role of vitamin D and calcium-vitamin D deficiency, vitamin D insufficiency and vitamin D sufficiency. Age Ageing 2000;29:301-4.
5. Kerstetter JE, Looker AC, Insogna KL. Low dietary protein and low bone density. Calcif Tissue Int 2000; 66:313.
6. Hegarty VM, May HM, Khaw KT. Tea drinking and bone mineral density in older women. Am J Clin Nutr 2000;71:1003-7.
7. Pfeifer M, Begerow B, Minne HW, et al. Effects of a short-term vitamin D and calcium supplementation on body sway and secondary hyperparathyroidism in elderly women. J Bone Mineral Res 2000;15:1113-8.
8. Weinsier RL, Krumdieck CL. Dairy foods and bone health: examination of the evidence. Am J Clin Nutr 2000;72:681-9 [review].

9. Brot C, Jørgensen N, Madsen O.R., Jensen L.B. & Sørensen O.H. Relationships between bone mineral density, serum vitamin D metabolites and calcium: phosphorus intake in healthy perimenopausal women. Journal of Internal Medicine Vol. 245 Issue 5 pgs 509-516.

10. Villareal DT, Holloszy JO, Kohrt WM.Effects of DHEA replacement on bone mineral density and body composition in elderly women and men. Clin Endocrinol (Oxf) 2000;53:561-8.

11. Adams JS, Kantorovich V, Wu C, et al. Resolution of vitamin D insufficiency in osteopenic patients results in rapid recovery of bone mineral density. J Clin Endocrinol Metab 1999;84:2729-30.

12. Salamone LM, Cauley JA, Black DM, et al. Effect of a lifestyle intervention on bone mineral density in premenopausal women: a randomized trial. Am J Clin Nutr 1999;70:97-103.

13. Rulm LA, Sakhaee K, Peterson R, et al. The effect of calcium citrate on bone density in the early and mid-postmenopausal period: a randomized, placebo-controlled study. Am J Ther 1999;6:303-11.

14. Leonetti HB, Longo S, Anasti JM. Transdermal progesterone cream for vasomotor symptoms and postmenopausal bone loss. Obstet Gynecol 1999;94:225-8.

15. Droisy R, Collette J, Chevallier T, et al. Effects of two 1-year calcium and vitamin D3 treatments on bone remodeling markers and femoral bone density in elderly women. Curr Ther Res 1998;59:850-62.

16. Lau EMC, Kwok T, Woo J, Ho SC. Bone mineral density in Chinese elderly female vegetarians, vegans, lacto-vegetarians and omnivores. Eur J Clin Nutr 1998;52:60-4.

17. Evans CE, Chughtai AY, Blumsohn A, et al. The effect of dietary sodium on calcium metabolism in premenopausal and postmenopausal women. Eur J Clin Nutr 1997;51:394-9.

18. Kim SH, Morton DJ, Barrett-Connor EL. Carbonated beverage consumption and bone mineral density among older women: the Rancho Bernardo Study. Am J Public Health 1997;87:276-9.

19. Owusu W, Willett WC, Feskanich D, et al. Calcium intake and the incidence of forearm and hip fractures among men. J Nutr 1997;127:1782-7.

20. Reid IR, Ames RW, Evans MC, et al. Long-term effects of calcium supplementation on bone loss and fractures in postmenopausal women: a randomized controlled trial. Am J Med 1995;98:331-5.

21. Strause L, Saltman P, Smith KT, et al. Spinal bone loss in postmenopausal women supplemented with calcium and trace minerals. J Nutr 1994;124:1060-4.

22. Gaby AR. Preventing and Reversing Osteoporosis. Rocklin, CA: Prima Publishing, 1994, 88-9 [review].

23. Heaney RP. Nutrient interactions and the calcium requirement. J Lab Clin Med 1994;124:15-6 [editorial/review].

24. Abraham GE, Grewal H. A total dietary program emphasizing magnesium instead of calcium. J Reprod Med 1990;35:503-7.

25. Prior JC. Progesterone as a bone-trophic hormone. Endocr Rev 1990;11:386-98.

26. Lee JR. Osteoporosis reversal: the role of progesterone. Int Clin Nutr Rev 1990;10:384-91.

27. Riis BJ, Thomsen K, Strom V, Christiansen C. The effect of percutaneous estradiol and natural progesterone on postmenopausal bone loss. Am J Obstet Gynecol 1987;156:61-5.

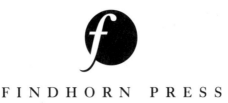

FINDHORN PRESS

Books, Card Sets,
CDs & DVDs
that inspire and uplift

For a complete catalogue,
please contact

Findhorn Press Ltd
305a The Park, Findhorn
Forres IV36 3TE
Scotland, UK

t +44(0)1309 690582
f +44(0)131 777 2711
e info@findhornpress.com

or consult our catalogue online
(with secure order facility) on
www.findhornpress.com

For information on the Findhorn Foundation:
www.findhorn.org